Testimonials

'I went to Dr (TCM) D'Alberto immediately after my third miscarriage, feeling very low and willing to try anything. My body was completely shattered, having been put through so much in a relatively short period of time. I asked Dr (TCM) D'Alberto how long it generally took people's bodies to get to the stage where they could consider IVF. He advised me the average time was six months, but that it would probably take longer for me due to the fact my body had gone through so much. Six months following my first consultation I found out I was pregnant naturally with our much-longed-for baby. With our history we hadn't expected to conceive naturally, and certainly not in such a short period of time! Due to my previous miscarriages I continued seeing Dr (TCM) D'Alberto throughout my pregnancy. I sailed through the pregnancy, and am now an extremely happy mummy to a four-month-old!.'

Mrs K

'On my journey I came across Dr (TCM) D'Alberto's website and contacted him right away. My first appointment with Attilio really impressed me; he asked questions and took notes to work out what might be the problem so he could decide which course of action to take. I left that session feeling very hopeful and with some reasons why I had issues getting pregnant. I left the clinic with a dietary plan and off I went to eat all the foods suggested for me *and follow my cycle. After eating the foods and acupuncture treatments, on day 13 I felt different – I felt tired and there were other little signs that I might be pregnant. By day 18 I was able to test and I was pregnant! My husband and I were so happy. I truly believe we got pregnant so quickly and easily after starting treatment with Attilio because of the acupuncture treatment and dietary advice recommended specifically for my needs. I had a very healthy pregnancy and continued to be very active. I had a natural birth with no complications. My baby is now four months old. I can't thank Attilio enough for his help achieving my dream of becoming a mummy.'*

Mrs C

'I started seeing Attilio for treatment after suffering a miscarriage and then finding out I was polycystic on one ovary. I had been trying to conceive for a number of months after the miscarriage and was starting to get very stressed and overwhelmed about the situation. After my initial consultation with Attilio I immediately felt calmer and more in control of my fertility. I started having weekly treatment and after completing only four sessions (one full cycle) I was astounded to find out I was pregnant! I had treatment until 20 weeks, and then again from 35 weeks to prepare me for labour. After a textbook pregnancy, I am now a very proud mum to a beautiful baby girl! Without Attilio's help I wouldn't have been blessed with my daughter.'

Mrs B

'I had been trying to conceive for two years when I approached Attilio. I was told by a fertility clinic that my hormone levels were too high and that I was approaching an early menopause. I was 41. I had had acupuncture in the past and knew how effective it could be, but I had never tried Chinese herbs and had heard they could lower hormone levels. Attilio diagnosed me as being blood and yin deficient – this explained my poor circulation, cracked tongue and general well-being. After six months of treatment with herbs and acupuncture and a diet to suit my condition, I am happy to say that my hormone levels returned to normal and I conceived naturally.'

Mrs J

'After four years of trying to conceive and being told that our only hope was IVF we took the advice of some friends to try acupuncture and Chinese medicine. Wow, what a piece of advice! Despite doctors performing numerous operations, they could only tell us it was unexplained infertility, and yet Attilio diagnosed our problem the moment we walked through the door! We had a sum total of six weeks of treatment with Attilio before falling pregnant, and have continued the treatment to ensure a healthy pregnancy. Having fertility problems is quite an emotional and private experience. However, since seeing Attilio we have been shouting about it from the rooftops and would thoroughly recommend that everyone try just one session, as that is all that is required to start seeing the benefits!'
Mr and Mrs T

'When I was told that my husband and I faced fertility problems I researched various possibilities of how I could affect them myself without jumping straight down the IVF route. I made some enquiries about Chinese herbal medicine and spoke to a few practitioners and decided to have an initial meeting with Attilio. Right from the start Attilio could read me like a book – he could tell me how I was feeling by my complexion and the colour of my tongue, and each week he would change my mix of herbs depending on how tired or busy I was. Five weeks later I was not only pregnant but also a lingering digestive problem had gone away.'
Ms L

'My husband and I have been trying for a baby for six years. After many tests, procedures and one miscarriage, we were told by doctors that we had "unexplained infertility" and our only option would be IVF. We decided to take their advice and began the rollercoaster that is IVF. Unfortunately the first cycle didn't work and we were gearing ourselves up for a second go when I came across Dr (TCM) D'Alberto. We met him and at our first meeting he said I had a yin and blood deficiency, which when we talked about it, made sense of everything – poor circulation and tiredness, to name but a few. We started a course of acupuncture and a new diet and within a couple of weeks I really had noticed a difference. Then, to my surprise, within six weeks I found out I was pregnant! I cannot tell you how excited we were and how grateful we are to Dr (TCM) D'Alberto. He also helped me over the first 12 weeks of my pregnancy when I was sick day and night and felt awful. I really don't know what I would have done without him.'

Mrs M

My Fertility Guide

How to get pregnant naturally

Dr (TCM) Attilio D'Alberto

www.attiliodalberto.com
www.myfertilityforum.com

To my partner Jamila and our little miracle Elisa

Contents

Introduction

Struggling to have a baby is a very personal and emotional problem, and is something that is not often shared with friends or even relatives. For this reason, it can feel like a lonely journey. If this sounds like you, then please rest assured that you are not alone. It is estimated that 1 in 6 couples in Western countries experience fertility challenges and this number is growing [1]. More and more couples are finding it difficult to have a baby and half of women struggling with fertility issues find it the most stressful experience of their lives [2].

A lot of women are now looking to start a family later in life. This is usually after they have built up their career, saved a deposit for a property and finally found a partner. At this point, mentally and emotionally, many women are in a better place to settle down and have a child. It can therefore come as a real shock to find that their body may have become weaker and is struggling to conceive and maintain a pregnancy.

If you're reading this book then you've most likely tried the natural route but still haven't had a baby. We all want the natural route to work and find it hard to accept when it doesn't. It can feel as though our bodies have forsaken us at a point in our lives when we are emotionally ready to have a child. This is where couples, and most often women, start to project-manage their fertility treatment and decide what to do next.

The guidance within this book can greatly increase your chances of having a baby naturally. For some couples this will be enough. Others may need a helping hand with acupuncture and Chinese herbs and some will need even more help by using assisted reproductive technologies, such as in-vitro fertilisation (IVF).

The length of time couples try to conceive naturally varies. For some it can be a few months and for others it's a few years. It's a personal choice. Until you fall pregnant, it can often feel like the rest of your life is on hold, with events such as holidays and weddings delayed until pregnancy is achieved. This focus and pressure can negatively affect fertility by causing frustration and stress, which can impact the normal balance of hormones within the body.

After trying naturally for a period of time, couples often make the decision to jump to IVF in an effort to conceive and get their lives back. IVF offers a 'process' – a start and an end with a projected success rate. It's this that attracts most couples to IVF, as trying naturally can seem like it's open-ended. However, due to the side effects of IVF [3], it should only be used as a last resort.

How this book can help you

One of the main reasons for writing this book is the lack of complete information available in one place, which means individuals have to scour the Internet and forums, piecing together different and sometimes contradictory bits of information, to compile a definitive understanding of conception. However, this can result in couples making the wrong decisions which wastes both time and money and causes stress, not to mention still leaving them without a baby.

In my experience with patients I've found that women are very knowledgeable about their fertility and require a lot more in-depth information than is often provided on websites or in other fertility books. I've therefore tried my best to include as much detailed information as possible in this book, but in a concise and easy-to-understand way. If you feel I can improve this book in any way, please do visit my website (**www.attiliodalberto.com**) and leave me some feedback.

There is around a 30 per cent chance of falling pregnant naturally each month [4]. There are three main problems that most couples have when trying for a baby – understanding:

1. how their body works
2. how to improve their lifestyle
3. how to optimise their diet

Within this book I will teach you how to increase your chances of having your baby. I will show you how to be more aware of your body, how to improve your lifestyle and outline diet plans for both you and your partner, together with supplements to take. I will explain the menstrual cycle and when it's best to try to conceive. I will also tell you which factors can affect male and female fertility and how to avoid them, how to improve egg and sperm quality, and aid implantation of the embryo into the uterus wall. I will also advise you on how to further support your natural fertility route.

Different couples are on different paths along their fertility journey; there are those who are just starting out and are finding it difficult to conceive and those who have been struggling for many years. This book caters for all couples who are trying naturally and need a little help. By prepping your body before conceiving, you are not only improving your health and your fertility but also helping your future child be in the best health possible for growth and development.

You can get additional support from the book's forum **www.myfertilityforum.com**, where we host a range of forums for women seeking advice, wanting to make new fertility friends and grow their support network.

About the author

I've been practising since 2004, using acupuncture and Chinese herbs to treat infertility. During this time, I've treated all types of infertility problems – for example unexplained infertility, endometriosis, low ovarian reserve, poor sperm motility and reoccurring miscarriages – for couples in their early twenties through to those in their late forties.

My studies in acupuncture and Chinese herbal medicine started a long time ago, with a five-year full-time degree programme in Traditional Chinese Medicine jointly run by Middlesex University in London and Beijing University of Traditional Chinese Medicine in China. Since graduating I've had numerous articles published in medical journals and healthcare magazines in various languages. I've learnt from some of the best acupuncturists in the world and now coach and advise other Chinese medicine practitioners.

I am passionate about acupuncture and Chinese medicine, the awareness it gives me and how I can use this to show people how to improve their health and have a baby. I blend ancient theories of Chinese medicine with modern scientific research to give a deeper insight into illness and disharmony, and then employ several treatment strategies to tackle the problem creating a higher success rate.

I believe it's important to explain to people what's going on with them and the disharmony they have, as it empowers them. This allows us to work consciously together to improve their chances of having a baby.

This book contains a lot of in-depth information which will greatly increase your chances of having a natural conception. By following my simple advice you too can fall pregnant naturally like the thousands of people I have treated.

Part One

Understanding the Fundamentals of Fertility

Before we get into the nitty-gritty of when you should be having sex to conceive a baby, it helps to first understand how your hormones work. By understanding them, you can see how making positive changes to your lifestyle and diet can greatly impact your hormones and your fertility.

Chapter 1

Your Hormones

Hormones are vital for health and fertility. Together they act like an orchestra, performing a symphony of bodily functions. The body is incredibly interconnected with many processes acting like a chain reaction. When they are performing in tune, fertility is balanced and harmonised. However, when they are performing out of tune, there is imbalance and infertility. Acupuncture acts like a conductor, helping to regulate and balance hormones so they work together in harmony.

It is very useful to have your hormones tested when you are trying to conceive as it gives you a valuable insight into what's going on inside your body. Hormone tests are valid for around three to four months. After that, new tests should be taken as the body is always changing and your hormone levels may have changed too. The range of a normal hormone level is constantly changing and can vary from clinic to clinic. Therefore, you might find the ranges within this book slightly different to yours.

Struggling with infertility can be stressful, emotional and draining. Stress and other factors create hormonal imbalances that can negatively impact fertility. From a Western medical point of view, stress can cause people to produce excessive cortisol, the stress hormone. This causes the body to use up important resources as well as affect an embryo implanting into the uterus wall [6]. Research has shown that women who start fertility treatment with too much cortisol in their body, have a reduced success rate [5]. The same applies to trying naturally. It's therefore important when trying naturally for a baby to reduce levels of cortisol. Research has shown that acupuncture reduces stress by regulating hormone levels [6]. Exercise can also help to reduce levels of cortisol within the body.

Let's now look at the array of different hormones that make up the orchestra of harmony within our bodies.

Hypothalamus Hormones

The hypothalamus is a major player in the body's orchestra and sets the scene for other organs that are linked to it, such as the pituitary gland. The hypothalamus is responsible for two major areas of survival: energy regulation and reproduction. When the body has better energy regulation, reproduction is better regulated. The hypothalamus produces gonadotrophin-releasing hormone (GnRH) and thyrotrophin-releasing hormone (TRH), which control the pituitary gland.

Gonadotrophin-releasing hormone (GnRH)

GnRH is produced from the hypothalamus and causes the pituitary gland to produce follicle stimulating hormone (FSH) and luteinising hormone (LH). Changes in the levels of GnRH are controlled by the amount of oestrogens (oestradiol), leptin and progestins (progesterone) in the blood. Oestrogens and leptin increase GnRH levels while progesterone decreases it. Research has shown that acupuncture is able to control GnRH thereby regulating the pituitary gland and its release of these fertility hormones [7] [8], thus improving female fertility.

Thyrotrophin-releasing hormone (TRH)

TRH is produced from the hypothalamus and causes the pituitary gland to produce thyroid stimulating hormone (TSH).

Pituitary Hormones

Let's now look at the next major organ involved in fertility: the pituitary gland. The pituitary gland produces several hormones. The important ones in fertility are FSH, LH, oxytocin, prolactin and TSH.

Follicle stimulating hormone (FSH)

FSH is produced by the pituitary gland after receiving the command from the hypothalamus. FSH is an important indicator of fertility. FSH stimulates the ovaries to grow multiple follicles – between 10 and 20 each month – all of which contain potential eggs. As one follicle becomes the biggest and matures, it releases oestradiol while the other follicles die off. The normal level of FSH is 3.5–12.5IU/mL on day 2–3 of your menstrual cycle. The level of FSH increases with age (see table below).

Age	FSH Level (IU/mL)
25–29	5–6
30–35	7–8
36–40	9–12
41–43	12–15

Table 1. Age-related FSH levels [9] [10]

FSH nourishes and grows the egg. Any physical deficiencies, such as a lack of energy, blood, lipids, protein and complex carbohydrates, that exist in the woman during the 85 days it takes for the egg to develop can affect its growth and maturation.

Research has shown that exposure to a cold environment can delay follicle growth and cause a low response of the ovaries to FSH [11]. FSH is made in the pituitary gland and shipped to the ovaries via the blood. To use an analogy, when it's cold outside and the roads are icy, transportation of goods from factories to the retail stores slows down. The same happens with the transportation of your FSH from the pituitary gland to the ovaries. Blood is a liquid and is affected by the cold. It slows down when it is cold, which means less FSH reaches the ovaries to stimulate egg growth. It is therefore important to keep your body warm and insulate it from the cold to keep the logistics of your body working properly.

Luteinising hormone (LH)

LH is produced during the daytime by the pituitary gland under direction from both the hypothalamus and the follicle [12]. As the follicle grows it releases oestrogens, which sends signals to produce LH to make it ripen and mature.

When LH surges, it triggers the final maturation of the follicle that contains the egg, the rupture of the follicle wall and the subsequent release of the egg into the fallopian tube. Levels of LH increase to between 21.9-56.6IU/mL.

The pituitary gland releases LH as a pulse. This pulse does not occur all the time, instead it happens in intervals. Ovulation kits use this surge in LH to determine ovulation. However, as LH is released in intervals, the time when the ovulation kit is used could potentially miss the pulse of the LH surge, thereby giving a false negative reading [13].

When a woman is fasting, levels of LH drop, which can affect ovulation [14]. This can be a problem for women who fast for weight loss or religious purposes. The normal level of LH is 2.1–12.6IU/mL on day 2-3 of your menstrual cycle. After ovulation, LH helps to maintain the empty follicle sac (corpus luteum), which in turn produces progesterone that maintains the uterus lining.

Oxytocin

Oxytocin is often known as the 'hug hormone', as physical contact increases its levels. It is released by the pituitary gland and is important for social behaviour, bonding, appetite, regulating anxiety, labour, lactation and in autism (people on the autism spectrum can have less oxytocin).

In men oxytocin helps to facilitate erectile function. Its levels increase during sexual intercourse and peak at orgasm, thereby aiding the transportation of sperm in the woman. In women oxytocin affects the uterus during labour by enhancing contractions of the muscles in the uterus wall, which push the baby out. After delivery, oxytocin helps to stimulate the release of milk (not its actual production) from the mother's breast.

A high-fat diet is associated with low levels of oxytocin [15]. Low levels of oxytocin make us feel more emotionally down and make us more likely to comfort eat, while high levels of oxytocin make us feel less hungry [16] [17]. Foods that are high in fat and sugar give us a feel-good factor (dopamine), but can make people put on weight. This weight gain can affect insulin levels, causing a rise in testosterone levels. High levels of testosterone commonly reduce levels of oxytocin, thus creating a vicious cycle.

Maintaining good levels of oxytocin is important not only for good health but also for good male and female fertility. Levels of oxytocin increase through physical contact, i.e. a hug or a massage from a partner, sexual intercourse or via acupuncture [18].

Prolactin

Prolactin is made by the pituitary gland. It stimulates a woman's breasts to develop and maintains the release of milk, hence 'lactin' relates to lactation. It also stops the menstrual cycle for the first few months after delivery, preventing another pregnancy [22]. A new mother is busy looking after and breastfeeding her newborn baby and does not have enough energy and blood to generate a menstrual cycle or grow another baby and placenta.

Prolactin is often measured in an initial hormone test along with oestrogens, FSH and TSH. The normal range of prolactin is between 2-29ng/mL on day 3 of the menstrual cycle. Levels of prolactin rise sharply during pregnancy. Otherwise, high levels of prolactin are sometimes seen in women with polycystic ovary syndrome (PCOS), hypothyroidism (underactive thyroid) and those who are stressed. Stress stimulates the pituitary gland to increase production of prolactin [19], which can cause an irregular menstrual cycle and infertility.

Thyroid stimulating hormone (TSH)

TSH triggers the release of thyroid hormones by the thyroid gland. The thyroid hormones it produces are thyroxine (T_4), triiodothyronine (T_3) and calcitonin (CT). The normal range for TSH is 0.2–4.0mU/L. However, for optimal fertility, the TSH level should be below 2.5mU/L. Some women may need to take drugs such as levothyroxine (thyroxine) to reduce their TSH level below 2.5mU/L even though it's still within the 'normal' range. Supplements such as iron and calcium can affect the absorption of levothyroxine, keeping TSH levels high. I therefore recommend not taking these supplements at the same time as levothyroxine. Instead, space them out to each end of the day, i.e. take one lot in the morning and the other lot in the evening time [20] [21].

Irregular levels of these hormones can directly affect fertility by causing the pituitary gland to increase the production of prolactin and decrease the production of FSH and LH, causing infertility.

During the menstrual cycle, levels of thyroid hormones fluctuate in relation to circulating levels of oestrogens. T_3 leads to a greater conversion of pregnenolone to progesterone. Women with an underactive thyroid tend to have lower levels of T_3, which lead to low levels of progesterone in the second half of their menstrual cycle. This may cause problems with the uterus lining and implantation.

Ovary Hormones

The ovaries produce follicles, which produce oestrogens and anti-Müllerian hormone (AMH). When ovulation has taken place, the empty follicle that once held the egg starts producing progesterone.

Once you are pregnant, the fertilised embryo releases the hormone human chorionic gonadotropin (hCG), which pregnancy tests detect to tell you that you are pregnant.

Oestrogens

Oestrogens are vital for a variety of bodily functions. In fertility their main functions are to maintain libido and female reproductive glands and organs, for example cervical mucous, as well as repair and regenerate the uterus (uterine-endometrial) lining. Oestrogens are made up of three hormones: oestradiol, oestrone and oestriol. The most abundant, and therefore the most important one for fertility, is oestradiol (also known as 17 beta-oestradiol or E2).

The normal level of oestradiol is 45–850pmol/L (12–230pg/mL) in the first part of your menstrual cycle (follicular phase). Higher than normal levels of oestradiol, greater than 290pmol/L (80pg/mL), can affect a fertilised embryo implanting into the uterus wall and mask a high FSH level [22]. Unfortunately, in the modern world we are all overdosing on man-made oestrogen (see page 59 for more on this). It's believed that the dramatic reduction in male and female fertility is due to excessive amounts of man-made oestrogens in the environment.

Anti-Müllerian hormone (AMH)

AMH has become a more accurate indicator of fertility in recent years replacing FSH. It is a measure of ovarian potential – how many eggs a woman has left in her body. However, it isn't a measure of egg quality. By measuring AMH levels, it helps to give perspective on a woman's fertility; a bit like looking inside the body to see what time the biological clock says. It can help to make better decisions when it comes to the changes that may be needed in order to have a baby and the treatment options available. AMH can be measured anywhere in the menstrual cycle from a blood test, but recent research has shown that AMH levels are slightly higher in the first part of the cycle before ovulation [23].

AMH is measured in either ng (nanogram) or pmol (picomole). Both levels are shown in the table below. These levels are constantly changing so they may differ to those in your country and clinic.

Level	ng/mL	pmol/L
Optimal fertility	12.7–21.6	28.6–48.5
Satisfactory fertility	7–12.7	15.7–28.5
Low fertility	1–6.9	2.2–15.6
Very low fertility	<1	<2.2

Table 2. AMH levels and ovarian potential

Unfortunately, AMH decreases with age. One study measured the AMH of 17,120 women in the United States [24]. The results are shown in table 3. This should help to give you a guide of what your AMH level should be for your age, although it is important to note that it is not definitive. As you can see, levels of AMH start to drop considerably from the age of 35 and then again at 41. Don't be alarmed by the drop in levels of AMH for your age. It only takes one good-quality egg to have a baby and I have helped women with an AMH of 1pmol/L fall pregnant naturally.

Low AMH levels can affect fertility. AMH can be seen as a measure of underlying fertility – what's left after years of living. However, by using the advice and guidance within this book over the 85-day period it takes for eggs to develop, it is possible to improve your egg quality enough for natural conception to take place and a healthy baby to be born.

Recent research has shown that women who are exposed to smoke from cigarettes and the burning of fuel, such as wood, can have reduced levels of AMH [25]. High AMH levels are sometimes seen in women with PCOS. The increase in the number of follicles on the ovaries causes an increase in levels of AMH, as each follicle releases AMH as well as oestrogens. Recent research has shown that acupuncture can reduce and normalise high AMH levels in women with PCOS [26] [27].

Age	ng/mL	pmol/L
26	4.2	30
27	3.7	26.4
28	3.8	27.1
29	3.5	25
30	3.2	22.8
31	3.1	22.1
32	2.5	17.9
33	2.6	18.6
34	2.3	16.4
35	2.1	15
36	1.8	12.9
37	1.6	11.4
38	1.4	10
39	1.3	9.3
40	1.1	7.9
41	1	7.1
42	0.9	6.4
43	0.7	5
44	0.6	4.3
45	0.5	3.6
46	0.4	2.9
47	0.4	2.9
48	0.2	1.4
49	0.1	0.7

Table 3. AMH levels in relation to age [24]

Progestins

Progestins, known as progestogens, are a group of steroid hormones produced by the corpus luteum (the sac that once held the egg) after ovulation. The most important progestin is progesterone, also known as P4. Progesterone has several important functions, including:

- Thickening the uterus lining.
- Propelling the egg along the fallopian tube.
- Aiding implantation.
- Enlarging the breasts.
- Maintaining the pregnancy.

New research has shown that progesterone aids in the production of TH2 cells (part of the immune system), which protect an implanting embryo [28]. It also induces lymphocytes (see page 52) to release an immunomodulatory protein that enhances TH2 production, both of which are needed for successful implantation [29].

The normal level of progesterone on day 3 of the menstrual cycle is less than 1nmol/L (0.31ng/mL). Progesterone production begins roughly 24 hours after ovulation – around day 15–16 on a normal 28–29.5-day cycle – and rises rapidly to a maximum 3–4 days after ovulation. The progesterone level at this time should be greater than 30nmol/L (9.43ng/mL), which indicates that ovulation has occurred. If conception does not occur, the corpus luteum disintegrates and progesterone levels fall, causing the start of the menstrual bleed. If conception does take place, the corpus luteum continues to produce progesterone until the placenta takes over from around weeks 8–12.

Human chorionic gonadotrophin (hCG)

The fertilised embryo produces hCG soon after it has implanted into the uterus wall [30]. hCG sustains the corpus luteum (the sac that contained the egg) for a further 3–4 months, thereby maintaining the production of progesterone. The testing of hCG levels in a woman's urine is how a home pregnancy test works and shows you that you are pregnant.

Adrenals

The adrenal glands sit on top of the kidneys. The adrenals produce several hormones. The ones important for fertility are glucocorticoids and dehydroepiandrosterone (DHEA).

Glucocorticoids

Glucocorticoids are made up of a group of hormones: cortisol (the most abundant of the three), corticosterone and cortisone. The hypothalamus sends corticotrophin-releasing hormone (CRH) to the pituitary gland, causing it to release adrenocorticotrophic hormone (ACTH), which stimulates the adrenals to produce cortisol, corticosterone and cortisone.

This group of hormones affects glucose levels, especially in the liver. These hormones are more present in times of stress and their effects are greater upon the liver. This is the same in Chinese medicine, where frustration (stress) affects the liver.

The body has three levels of stress response:
1. The alarm phase (level 1).
2. The resistance phase (level 2).
3. The exhaustion phase (level 3) [30].

Prolonged stress (for more than a few hours), which includes starvation (dieting) and anxiety, causes the body to go into the resistance phase (level 2). Most people live in the resistance phase causing the production of ACTH and the release of glucocorticoids, which uses up energy, lipids and proteins, and can cause a stressed liver, which leads to higher levels of cortisone, irregular levels of fertility hormones and infertility.

Dehydroepiandrosterone (DHEA)

DHEA is a 'parent hormone' in that it creates other hormones. It is mainly produced by the adrenal glands. In men, DHEA is also produced by the testes. It is changed in the body to a hormone called androstenedione. Androstenedione is then changed into the major male and female hormones: testosterone and oestrogens.

In women with low AMH levels and poor egg quality, DHEA might be useful. In one study, taking DHEA (75mg) six weeks prior to starting an IVF cycle increased the quantity of eggs collected, increased egg quality and improved the live birth rate [31]. Further studies have shown that taking DHEA (25mg) in conjunction with coenzyme q10 (600mg) increased egg quality [32]. Other studies that tested DHEA at various dosages have found it to be effective for fertility [33] [34] (see page 189 for more on DHEA).

The Liver

The liver produces sex hormone-binding globulin (SHBG), which regulates testosterone levels in the body.

Sex hormone-binding globulin

Sex hormone-binding globulin (SHBG) is a carrier protein that binds to testosterone. The normal range of SHBG is 18–114nmol/L on day 3 of the menstrual cycle. Testosterone that is bound to SHBG is unable to bind to testosterone receptors and is inactive. Therefore, the more SHBG hormone that's in the body, the less free testosterone is available, which can affect follicle growth. Only a small fraction (1–3 per cent) of testosterone is unbound and free. It's this small per cent of free testosterone that exerts its effects upon the body and fertility.

The liver makes SHBG after receiving the message from oestrogens. High levels of oestrogens make the liver produce more SHBG, which leads to less free testosterone. This is one way in which the body balances its hormones. The liver lies at the cornerstone of acupuncture treatment for female infertility. By regulating the liver, the body is able to regulate levels of oestrogens and testosterone.

Women with a thyroid disorder can have unbalanced levels of SHBG and therefore abnormal testosterone levels. High levels of SHBG are characteristic of hyperthyroidism (overactive thyroid), which causes low levels of free testosterone, while low levels of SHBG are characteristic of hypothyroidism (underactive thyroid), which causes high levels of testosterone.

Multiple Hormone Sites

Hormones are made in various parts of the body, for example in the digestive system as well as in the reproductive organs.

Testosterone

Testosterone is the primary androgen that causes increased hair growth, acne and virilisation (the development of male characteristics). It is released by the adrenal glands (25 per cent) and the ovaries (25 per cent), and is produced in adipose (fat) tissue (50 per cent). Its production is dependent upon LH. If women are dieting or fasting, they will have lower levels of LH, which will lead to lower levels of testosterone.

There are two types of testosterone: one that is bound to SHBG and therefore inactive and another that is not bound and is therefore free and active. The latter type is the one that has an effect upon fertility. The normal level of active testosterone on day 3 of the menstrual cycle is 0.5–3.6nmol/L (14-103ng/dL). In men, testosterone helps with sperm production. In females, it aids follicle growth, but too much can cause PCOS.

The Pancreas

The pancreas has similar functions to the spleen in Chinese medicine. It produces insulin, which regulates glucose in the body. In Chinese medicine, the flavour attributed to the spleen is sweet. A heavy meal often weakens the spleen and pancreas, hence why people tend to crave a sweet pudding afterwards, to help aid spleen and pancreas function, thereby improving digestion.

Insulin

Insulin is a hormone produced by the pancreas that decreases levels of glucose in the blood. The more sugar that's in the body, the higher the level of insulin, which can lead to type 2 diabetes. Glucose is a type of sugar. The normal level of insulin should be less than 7.8mmol/L (140mg/dL). Insulin stimulates fat storage [35]. Women who are overweight tend to have higher levels of insulin, caused by eating too much sugar or fat, and low levels of oxytocin circulating in their blood.

Insulin reduces the levels of SHBG, causing more circulating testosterone and LH in the body, leading to infertility and possibly PCOS [35]. Women who are underweight tend to have lower levels of insulin that decreases the stimulation of the pituitary gland and the ovaries causing an irregular menstrual cycle and infertility [36].

Apart from sugar, insulin is also affected by stress. Research studies have demonstrated the effectiveness of acupuncture in regulating insulin levels as well as reducing stress [37]. Artificial sweeteners, which are used as a sugar substitute, are now believed to interfere with insulin levels and can actually cause weight gain [38].

Later in the book, I will discuss diet and how to optimise it to improve your fertility. I will also give you a diet plan which will help to reduce sugar levels that can affect implantation and optimise your hormones as well as strengthen your body.

Chapter 2

The Components of Fertility

Understanding the basic components of fertility allows us to home in on each aspect to optimise it for better fertility and natural conception. This should be done in conjunction with a broader view of overall general health, as explained later. Essentially, becoming pregnant can be broken down into three components: the quality of the egg and sperm, the sperm's journey to the egg and the receptibility of the uterus lining.

Follicles (eggs)

At birth, a woman will have between 500,000 and 1,000,000 follicles (each containing an egg). Incredibly, with a woman ovulating just once a month from puberty to menopause, fewer than 500 of the 500,000–1,000,000 eggs will reach ovulation [4] [30] [39]. During each menstrual cycle, around 10–20 follicles are stimulated at once with generally just one becoming dominant and ovulating. This number declines rapidly by the age of 38, with around 25,000 remaining in the ovaries, and then decreasing ever more rapidly until about 1000 remain around the age of menopause, normally around the age of 49.

Follicles are dependent upon good amounts of anti-Müllerian hormone (AMH) and androgens (testosterone, androstenedione and sex hormone-binding globulin (SHBG)). The follicle converts androgens into oestrogens, which helps it grow. The follicles also need good amounts of protein and complex carbohydrates to grow. It takes 85 days for the egg to grow from start to finish [40].

Uterus (uterine-endometrial) lining

A woman's uterus lining should be thick enough to allow an embryo to implant and grow, and shouldn't be hostile to implantation. At the start of the menstrual cycle, the uterus lining is thin, as the lining has shed causing the menstrual bleed. The release of oestrogens by the growing follicles causes the lining to thicken. The thickness reaches its peak at around day 21 in a 28-day menstrual cycle, when implantation of the fertilised embryo should be occurring.

As oestrogens surge, they repair and regenerate the uterus lining. The uterus lining will gradually thicken, reaching its maximum thickness around day 21 when implantation should take place. The minimal thickness is 7–8+mm with a triple lining (triple stripe). This triple lining is the three layers that make up the uterus wall (endometrium, myometrium and perimetrium).

More and more women are discovering their infertility is due to a hyperactive immune system in their uterus, where the immune system prevents the embryo implanting into the uterus wall. The reasons for this are complex, but can be due to stress, an irregular lifestyle, poor diet, a high intake of refined sugar and exposure to multiple chemicals, which I'll explain in Chapter Four.

Sperm

The volume of semen in a typical ejaculation is 2.5-5mL, with 50-150 million sperm per mL, giving an average normal sperm count of 125-750 million [39]. When trying for a baby, having sexual intercourse just around the time of ovulation sends billions of sperm on the hunt for one egg! However, only 1 per cent of sperm will reach the cervix and only around 0.01 per cent from each ejaculation will reach the ovary [39].

Sperm health has been plummeting since 1938 [41]. This is mainly caused by exposure to chemicals, excessive stress and poor lifestyle and diet choices. Making simple changes to a man's diet and lifestyle can have a massive positive impact upon his sperm quality, which we will cover in Chapters Seven, Eight, Nine and Ten.

Because the sperm need to travel a vast distance they must be strong and mobile. This journey from the vaginal canal up into the fallopian tube where insemination takes place helps to eliminate the weak from the strong and gives a higher probability that sperm with intact DNA in their head are able to reach the egg and penetrate it. However, the DNA within a mature sperm head can still have chromosome abnormalities. It's therefore important to try to improve sperm quality as much as possible.

Understanding the Menstrual Cycle

The word 'menstrual' comes from the Latin word for 'month' and the word 'month' comes from the Latin for 'moon'. This is the same in Chinese, where the Chinese character Yuè 月 relates to the menstrual cycle, month and moon [42]. Historically, it's believed that woman's menstrual cycle would have followed the lunar cycles. A normal menstrual cycle is around 28–29.5 days long, which follows the moon's length of cycle.

The menstrual cycle is made up of two sub-cycles: one for the ovaries and one for the uterus. Regulating and syncing both these cycles is key to good fertility. The main hormones involved in the ovary cycle are follicle stimulating hormone (FSH) and luteinising hormone (LH), while the main hormones involved in the uterus cycle are oestrogens (mainly oestradiol) and progestins (progesterone) – see Figure 3 (page 42).

Ovary cycle

The ovary cycle is made up of two phases: the follicular phase and the luteal phase (see Figure 3, page 42). The follicular phase starts with the menstrual bleed and is the maturing of a dominant follicle that contains the egg. The luteal phase starts with ovulation and is the release of the egg into the fallopian tube, insemination of the egg by a sperm, the moving of the egg down the fallopian tube and implantation of the fertilised egg into the uterus wall (uterine-endometrial lining) – see Figure 1 (page 38).

Uterus cycle

The uterus cycle involves the breakdown of the uterus lining, when a woman has her menstrual bleed at the beginning of the follicular phase and the building up of the uterus lining to its peak in the luteal phase.

Premenstrual symptoms, commonly perceived as normal, are actually indicators of problems with the menstrual cycle and therefore fertility [43]. Acupuncture is very good at treating premenstrual symptoms, regulating the menstrual cycle and problems with menstrual blood flow, thereby improving fertility [8] [7] [44].

At the start of a woman's menstrual cycle, the uterus lining sheds due to a lack of both oestrogens and progestins that are needed to sustain it, leaving only the base layer. A good period flow should last between five and seven days and be heavy for the first three to five days, then reduce to medium then light. Typically, a woman will lose 50–90ml of red blood without clots. If the blood is dark, is not heavy on day 1 or contains clots, it indicates a problem with the menstrual cycle and fertility.

As a menstrual bleed takes place, the hypothalamus releases gonadotropin-releasing hormone (GnRH), which initiates the pituitary gland to start the production of FSH. This in turn stimulates the ovaries to grow follicles.

Follicles sit in a procession known as an antral follicle count (AFC). The better the woman's health, the more follicles she will have and the better her egg quality will be. You can help increase your egg quality by making changes to your lifestyle and diet as outlined in Chapters Seven, Eight, Nine and Ten.

Between 10 and 20 follicles are stimulated in each menstrual cycle. As the follicles mature, one becomes dominant and releases oestrogens, while the others die off.

As oestrogen levels rise steeply, they increase the thickness of the uterus lining and start the production of LH. This helps the egg to ripen and eject from the follicle sac.

Ovulation

At around day 14–15 in a typical 28–29.5-day cycle, there is a massive release of LH from the pituitary gland. The LH surge begins 34–36 hours before ovulation and peaks 10–12 hours prior to the egg being released (see Figure 3, page 42) [13]. This LH surge is used by ovulation kits to test when it's the right time for couples to have sexual intercourse. The LH surge pulsates, so it's not continuous and therefore ovulation kits may not always detect the LH surge. I would recommend watching your body's own signs of ovulation (see below) instead of using ovulation kits, which are often expensive, inaccurate and can cause stress and disappointment.

The surge in LH causes the release of the egg from the ovary. At this point, the follicle is around 18–25mm in size and has reached maturation.

The high LH levels that trigger ovulation also maintain the sac that once held the egg, called the corpus luteum, and its production of the main progestin hormone progesterone, which maintains the uterus lining.

Progesterone production begins around 24 hours before ovulation [13]. Progesterone supports the flow of blood to the uterus lining, thereby maintaining it. It also increases the production of immune cells that aid implantation. Progesterone levels remain high for about a week and drop off if pregnancy is not achieved, causing the disintegration of the uterus lining and the menstrual bleed to begin.

Fertilisation and implantation

Once natural insemination takes place in the fallopian tube, the embryo will start to divide (cleavage). The first division starts 24 hours after fertilisation has taken place and is completed six hours later. Each succeeding division takes slightly less time. By the end of the second day there are four cells. By the end of the third day, there are 16 cells. By the end of the fifth day there are 32 cells and the embryo has formed into a blastocyst [39]. This all occurs as the fertilised embryo travels down your fallopian tube towards your uterus (see Figure 1, page 38).

Any blockages en route, for example scar tissue from surgery or an infection, may cause the fertilised egg to become lodged against the lining of the fallopian tube where it will start to grow, causing an ectopic pregnancy. This can be life-threatening for the woman. Once the fertilised egg (zygote) has reached the uterus, it will implant into the side of the uterus wall around six days after ovulation. The egg does this by burrowing a small hole into the uterus wall (see Figure 1, page 38). Some women will notice spotting or a pink discharge as the embryo releases blood while burrowing into the uterus wall, although this is uncommon.

Symptoms of an ectopic pregnancy
- Sharp pain in the abdomen which can radiate to the shoulder or neck.
- Chronic pain that occurs on one side of the abdomen.
- Heavy to light vaginal bleeding or spotting.
- Dizziness or fainting.
- Pain when defecating.

Once implantation has taken place, blood flow will quicken around the woman's body and to the uterus. Demands on the mother for energy and blood will greatly increase. This is why some women feel tired when they fall pregnant. The embryo starts to release the hormone human chorionic gonadotrophin (hCG), which is used by pregnancy tests to determine if you're pregnant. If the pregnancy test is very faint, a blood test can be used instead, which picks up low levels of hCG.

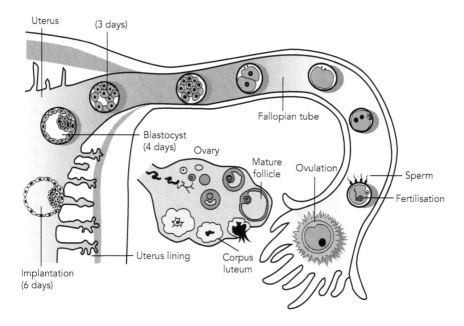

Figure 1. Fertilisation, journey and implantation of the embryo

Knowing When to Have Sex

Most women will ovulate mid-cycle, around day 14–15. For couples trying for a baby naturally it is ideal to have sexual intercourse 1–2 days before the LH surge as the sperm are able to wait next to the ovary for 48 hours until ovulation occurs. This will mean having sex on days 12–13. It can take between 30 minutes and two hours for the sperm to travel up into the cervix and into the fallopian tube where insemination takes place.

Midway through your menstrual cycle just before and during ovulation, you should have a stringy discharge that exits the vagina. This is known as cervical mucus as it drips down from the cervix. The sperm travel up into the cervix via the woman's cervical mucus discharge. It looks a bit like egg white and for that reason it's often referred to as that. You can check if you have this egg white discharge by taking some of it in your fingers and pulling it apart. It should stretch apart, unlike your normal discharge at other times in your cycle (see Figure 2 below). When you begin to notice this egg white discharge, you should start having sexual intercourse.

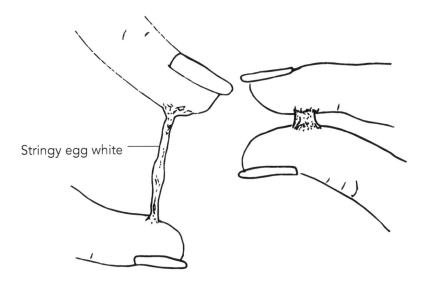

Stringy egg white

Figure 2. The stretching difference between cervical mucus (egg white) and normal vaginal discharge

If no cervical mucus exists, it could mean it is high up in the vaginal canal, that there isn't a lot, or there is none at all. An artificial substitute lube that mimics a woman's cervical mucus can be used to assist the sperms' travel into the cervix. This is applied to the woman's vagina before sexual intercourse and can be bought from most pharmacies. Once the sperm reach the ovary, they can wait and recharge for a few days until the egg is released.

Couples can start trying two-three days before ovulation and then once to twice a day until one day after ovulation to ensure they have covered all chances [39] [356]. Men should ejaculate 'old' sperm from their testis three days prior to sexual intercourse to ensure that only fresh, healthy sperm are used for conception. Fertilisation needs to take place 12–24 hours after the egg has been released from the ovary, so it's best to have sex before ovulation than afterwards. It is not advisable to try excessively at other times in the cycle as this can lead to male fertility problems, for example poor sperm quality caused by exhaustion of the body's resources.

Some women notice twinges and bloating a few days before they ovulate as the follicle swells inside them and puts pressure on surrounding structures. This is a good time to start trying. If the twinges are painful it may indicate cysts or polyps on the ovaries. In such cases, a scan is useful to identify any abnormalities. Some women may feel tired and crave sugar. It takes a lot of energy and resources to produce a good-quality egg every month. A woman's appetite can increase after ovulation, probably as a result of being physically depleted from ovulating [45]. Some women may get lower back pain or may feel dizzy or aren't as mentally alert as normal, which highlight a problem with their health and fertility. These symptoms can easily be rectified by making changes to your lifestyle and diet, as explained in Chapter Seven, Eight, Nine and Ten.

Charting

Body temperatures fluctuate throughout the menstrual cycle. The basal body temperature rises by 0.8–0.9°C after ovulation. This is caused by progesterone affecting the brain's thermo-regulator [13]. During ovulation, temperatures drop noticeably, and then rise sharply, making it possible to know when ovulation occurs if body temperatures are being recorded.

Otherwise known as 'charting' or 'BBT charting', some women in my clinic use this method to predict when they're ovulating and when to have sexual intercourse. It can also be used by holistic practitioners to gauge any problems with hormone levels in the menstrual cycle. However, in my opinion, charting can cause stress as temperatures need to be taken at the same time every morning, which doesn't allow for a lie in and is a constant reminder upon waking that fertility is an issue.

In my experience, charting can be useful for the first few months of trying to conceive. After a couple of month, some women can find it causes them stress. Stress is a big problem in fertility as it can make the menstrual cycle irregular and cause a hyperactive immune system, which affects implantation. Looking out for signs and symptoms of ovulation is less stressful and can be a more reliable method in determining ovulation. These signs and symptoms vary from woman to woman, but generally include:

- bloating
- discharge changes to thick and stringy (egg white)
- increased appetite
- increased libido
- twinges over the ovaries

Fertility apps

A lot of women are now using fertility apps on their smartphones to keep a track of their menstrual cycle and when they are going to ovulate and should have intercourse. These apps can be useful, but unfortunately, like charting, they can also increase stress levels, which can work against fertility [46].

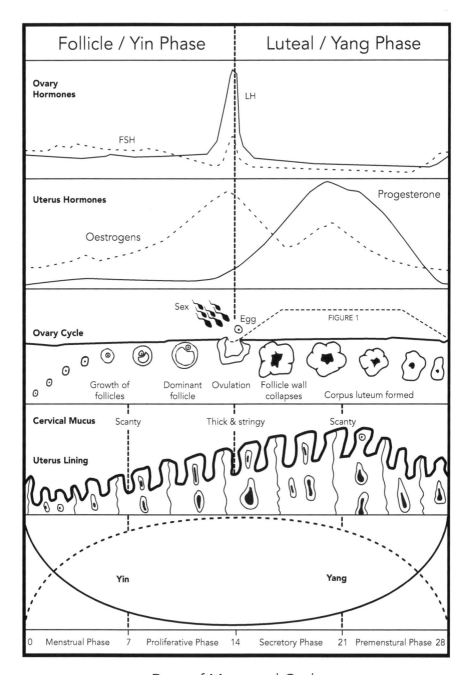

Days of Menstrual Cycle

Figure 3. The menstrual cycle and its hormones

Stages of the menstrual cycle and conception

Days 1–5

Progesterone levels are at their lowest level, which causes:

- Bleeding as the uterus lining is no longer maintained.
- The hypothalamus sends messages (GnRH) to the pituitary gland to start producing FSH to stimulate the growth of new follicles in the ovaries.

Days 6–7

- One of the follicles becomes dominant and starts producing large quantities of oestrogens, mainly oestradiol.

Days 8–13

- High levels of oestradiol stimulate:
  - the uterus lining to thicken
  - the glands in the cervix to produce mucus (egg white)
- Sexual intercourse together with the father's energy injects semen into the vagina where the sperm travel up into the cervix using the cervical mucus as a ladder.

Days 14–15

- The pituitary gland starts to produce LH, causing the egg to mature and rupture from the follicle.
- A sperm inseminates the egg.

Days 16–25

- The empty follicle sac is now called the corpus luteum and starts to produce progesterone, causing the thickening and maintaining of the uterus lining.
- The egg travels down the fallopian tube into the uterus.

Days 25–28

- The egg (now called a morula) arrives in the uterus four days later. Over the next 2–3 days it will form into a blastocyst and embed itself into the side of the uterus wall.

- If fertilisation doesn't take place, the corpus luteum disintegrates and progesterone levels drop, causing the start of bleeding and the next menstrual cycle.

Weeks 5–8

- The fertilised egg (now called a zygote) begins releasing hCG hormone, which maintains the corpus luteum and the production of progesterone until the placenta takes over.

- A pregnancy test picks up the hCG levels and the test is positive.

Table 4. Summary of the stages of the menstrual cycle and implantation

Chapter 3

Getting Your Fertility Tested

There are several tests that can be carried out (by your local doctor) to assess your fertility. The tests see if there are any blockages obstructing the sperm getting to the egg and if any hormone imbalances are preventing the normal workings of the ovary and uterus cycles.

Semen Test

The simplest and most painless fertility test is a semen analysis that a man can do at any time. It's best for the man to abstain from ejaculating three to four days prior to giving a sample. Once the sample has been given, it needs to reach the laboratory within 30 minutes [36].

The parameters for a semen sample are set by the World Health Organization (WHO) and are constantly being reviewed [47]. Some countries use the old parameters and some the new. According to the latest report (fifth version), a normal semen sample should be:

- Semen volume: more than 1.5mL.
- Sperm count: more than 39 million in total.
- Sperm concentration: more than 15 million per ml.
- Sperm motility (movement): more than 32 per cent moving.
- Sperm morphology (shape): more than 4 per cent of normal shape.

- Vitality (live sperm): more than 58 per cent.
- White blood cells: less than 1 million per ml.
- Anti-sperm antibodies test: should be negative.

These semen ranges are constantly being lowered as male fertility declines. This downward trend has been happening since the 1930s. Over a 40-year period, male sperm numbers have reduced by 60 per cent [48]. Large numbers of sperm – not just one – are needed for successful fertilisation. Many sperm are needed to attack and erode the outer layer of the egg (zona pellucida) allowing one sperm to enter. Therefore, if a man has a sperm count lower than 20 million, he is considered infertile as there aren't enough sperm that will reach the ovary and for fertilisation to occur [30].

There can be large differences in semen results, so the results of a single semen analysis should be not taken literally and another sample should be retested after three months. Higher counts are common during winter [49]. Before giving a sample, the penis and hands should be washed making sure all soap has been removed. No lubricating jelly should be used as this can kill the sperm, as can soap residue.

The act of a man masturbating in a strange room with a person, often a woman, waiting outside can cause stress and may affect the level of ejaculation and therefore the semen result. It's not a proper, love-filled, emotional and sensual ejaculation, but unfortunately there is no alternative. Home kits are available, though they don't give a complete analysis of semen quality.

It takes around 10–12 weeks for sperm to be developed. During this 10–12-week development period, sperm quality can be improved by making changes to the man's lifestyle and diet (see Chapters Seven, Eight, Nine and Ten for more on this).

Hormone and Measles Tests

The standard fertility tests that are conducted in women include:

- anti-Müllerian hormone (AMH)
- coagulation screening
- complete blood count
- follicle stimulating hormone (FSH)
- luteinising hormone (LH)
- oestrogens
- progesterone
- prolactin
- rhesus negative
- rubella (German measles, which can cause infertility and birth defects)
- thyroid stimulating hormone (TSH)

These are conducted from a blood test at the start of the menstrual cycle and are the basic set of tests. More complex tests, such as immune testing and chromosome analysis, can be carried out if couples have been struggling to conceive for some time (see page 52).

It is best to get these tests done on day 2 or 3 of your cycle, except for progesterone. A progesterone test is often taken on day 21 if it's a normal 28-day menstrual cycle. However, it's more accurate to measure progesterone seven days before the next bleed to determine whether ovulation has occurred.

Some women, for example those with PCOS, may need to have their testosterone levels measured. Some men may also need to have their testosterone and FSH levels checked depending on their individual health, age and semen result.

Uterus and Fallopian Tube Tests

There are several tests that can be conducted to see if a woman's uterus is the normal size and if the fallopian tubes are open or blocked.

The uterus should be 6–10cm in size. If the uterus is smaller than this (known as 'hypoplasia uterus') it can lead to lack of a menstrual cycle and infertility. Some uteruses can be angled differently or have different shapes, which can affect fertility. The fallopian tubes connect the ovaries to the uterus, like a funnel, and are where the sperm meets the egg and conception occurs. Having clear and open tubes is therefore very important for fertility. If a woman's fallopian tubes are blocked (tubal occlusion) by tissue or other bodily masses, it can obstruct the sperm getting to the egg, causing infertility. However, it's possible to unblock less chronic obstructions using acupuncture and Chinese herbs [50] or during an internal examination such as a Hysterosalpingo Contrast Sonography (HyCoSy) – see below.

The several tests that can be performed to check if your tubes are open are shown below. In most instances, it's best to have someone take you home from the clinic after the procedure as you may be drowsy from the sedative medication and be in some discomfort. If you have pain after the procedure, apply a hot water bottle to your abdomen and have acupuncture.

There is an increased chance of conceiving naturally after having your tubes check to see if they are open (tubal patency). This is because the solution that is injected into your fallopian tubes can flush out any blockages, allowing the sperm to reach the egg.

Hysterosalpingo Contrast Sonography (HyCoSy)

A speculum (an instrument to open your vagina) is inserted into your vagina, like a smear test, and your cervix (neck of your womb) is cleaned with an antiseptic solution. A small thin catheter (tube) is passed through the cervix into the uterus and a small balloon is inflated to keep the catheter in position. A vaginal ultrasound scan is carried out to locate the uterus and ovaries. Echo contrast fluid is inserted into the fallopian tubes via the catheter, to show up on the ultrasound scan as thin lines, which shows that your tubes are open.

Hysterosalpingo-Foam Sonography (HyFoSy)

A speculum is inserted into your vagina and your cervix is cleaned with an antiseptic solution. A fine catheter is passed through your cervix into your uterus, ready for the contrast solution of sterile water and sterile inert gel, which has been mixed together to create a foamy liquid. The solution is passed through the catheter while an internal vaginal scan is performed. The foamy solution should show as bright white on the screen, first filling your uterus, then showing as fine lines as it flows through your tubes, showing your tubes are open.

Hysterosalpingography (HSG)

A hysterosalpingography is also called a uterosalpingography. A fluid is inserted into the uterus and up into the fallopian tubes, then an X-ray is taken to check and see if the fluid is running into the fallopian tubes. It does not usually require a general anaesthetic. An HSG should be done within 10 days of a menstrual period starting. Pregnancy should be ruled out beforehand as the X-ray can affect the foetus.

Hysteroscopy

A hysteroscopy is a procedure where a special narrow telescope called a hysteroscope is passed through the vagina and cervix, into the uterus. No incisions are made. A biopsy will be taken from the uterus lining if any abnormalities are found, such as fibroids, polyps or endometrial tissue. It is also possible to take a biopsy with the woman awake, but on some occasions a general anaesthetic is used, depending on how uncomfortable and painful it is for the woman. This is usually carried out as a day case, although there is a chance the woman will need to stay in hospital overnight, especially if anything is found during the examination and treatment was carried out at the same time, for example the removal of a polyp.

Laparoscopy and dye test ('lap and dye')

A laparoscopy involves admission to hospital and is performed under a general anaesthetic. A small incision is made in the abdomen and a needle inserted. A telescope called a laparoscope is inserted into the abdomen. The uterus, tubes and ovaries are then examined. Dye is passed through the cervix into the uterus and fallopian tubes to show it flowing freely to the ovaries.

Other uterus tests include:

- Ultrasound: used to assess the size and shape of the uterus, its thickness and the number of follicles in each ovary (antral follicle count).

- Doppler ultrasound: the combination of an ultrasound with a Doppler measurement can give a useful look at follicle growth around the time of ovulation as well as being a non-invasive method of assessing blood flow to the uterus.

- Shape: the shape of the uterus can affect fertility. For example, a heart-shaped uterus (known as a 'bicornuate uterus') has a higher miscarriage and preterm labour rate. Other uterus shapes include: 'unicornuate', 'double' and 'septate' uteruses [4].

Around 20 per cent of women will have a uterus that bends backwards (called a 'retroflexion' or 'retroverted uterus'), which doesn't affect conceiving naturally. During the third trimester of pregnancy, a retroverted uterus can spontaneously correct its position.

Antral Follicle Count (AFC)

An AFC is used to see the number of follicles that are about to develop into potential eggs. It is often used as a measure of fertility and ovarian reserve in conjunction with an AMH test (see page 24). The follicles are viewed and then measured using an ultrasound. There will be varying sizes of follicles, some 2–6mm in diameter and others 7–10mm. Generally, there should be around a dozen, depending on the woman's health, fertility and age. The number of small follicles, called granulosa cells, measuring 2–6mm in diameter declines with age, while the larger 7–10mm size follicles doesn't. Research has shown that acupuncture is able to increase AFC levels [51]. Lifting heavy objects or working night shifts can decrease AFC levels and affect the menstrual cycle [12] [52] [53] [54]. This is especially true in women who are either overweight or over 37 years old. This is because both of these activities can deplete a woman's resources, which are used to generate a woman's eggs.

Sexually Transmitted Infections (STIs)

It is worth getting you and your partner checked for any STIs. Both chlamydia and gonorrhoea can cause infections in the pelvis (pelvic inflammatory disease), which may damage the fallopian tubes causing ectopic pregnancies, chronic pain and infertility. These tests can be done by your doctor or at a sexual health clinic and involve giving a blood, urine and swab samples.

Thrombophilia Test

A thrombophilia is a blood clot that can occur in the umbilical cord, blocking blood and nutrients reaching the growing baby, causing it to miscarry. The test looks for anticoagulant deficiencies that might cause a blood clot. Heparin (enoxaparin) is often given to women with a family history of thrombophilia [55]. Aspirin (acetylsalicylic acid) is commonly prescribed by doctors for blood clotting, but aspirin can greatly reduce melatonin levels, which can reduce egg and sperm quality.

Zika Virus

The Zika virus is transmitted sexually or via mosquito bites and causes congenital birth defects [56]. Zika is spread mostly by the bite of an infected *Aedes* species mosquito (*Ae. aegypti* and *Ae. albopictus*). These mosquitoes bite during the day and night. The most common symptoms are fever, rash, headache, joint pain, red eyes and muscle pain. If you've recently travelled to a place where the Zika virus is present you may need to get tested. Your doctor may order a blood or urine test to help determine if you have Zika. There is no specific medicine for Zika [57]. You should wait for at least two months after visiting a Zika virus country before trying to conceive a baby [58].

Chromosomal Analysis

A chromosomal analysis is sometimes performed for couples who've had repeated miscarriages. An abnormal foetal karyotype (number of chromosomes) is found in around 50–70 per cent of miscarriages [59]. Women are more affected by chromosome abnormalities than men [60]. For older women the risk of ovulating a chromosomally abnormal egg might be 50 per cent or higher [40] [59]. Improving egg quality (see Chapter Seven) can improve chromosomes.

Immune Testing

The immune system plays an important role in fertility. It mediates the embryo implanting into the uterus wall. If the embryo implants too deeply into the uterus wall, it can affect the mother's health, while too little can cause the embryo to miscarry.

Part of the immune system is made up of white blood cells. Around 20–30 per cent of these white blood cells are made up of lymphocytes. There are three types of lymphocytes:

1. T cells: responsible for cell-mediated immunity – our defence against abnormal cells and pathogens inside living cells.
2. B cells: responsible for antibody-mediated immunity – our defence against antigens and pathogenic organisms in body fluids.
3. Natural killer (NK) cells: attack foreign cells, normal cells infected with viruses and cancer cells.

Around 80 per cent of lymphocytes are T cells; 10–15 per cent are B cells and 5–10 per cent are NK cells.

There are two main types of NK cells: those circulating in the blood (pkNK) and those in the uterus (uNK). Within the blood, 90 per cent of pkNK cells are $CD56^{dim}CD16^+$ and 10 per cent are $CD56^{bright}CD16$, while in the uterus the main types of uNK cells are $CD56^{bright}$ and CD16 [61]. There is much debate amongst fertility experts and immunologists as to the importance of NK cells in fertility. It's known that NK cells help the embryo implant into the uterus wall [61]. However, some fertility experts believe that too many NK cells can impede implantation and should therefore be treated with strong drugs that suppress them.

B cells

B cells target antigens. Antigens are pathogens, parts of products of pathogens or other foreign compounds. These B cells use an immune hormone protein to communicate, called a cytokine. The cytokine is released by T helper cells (TH and CD4+) and triggers the activation of the B cells. B cells secrete antibodies that attack antigens.

CD4+ Th cell-mediated specific immune responses are made up of two forms: type 1 T helper (TH1) and type 2 T helper (TH2) cells. Both environmental and genetic factors act together to determine which one will be dominant, either TH1 or TH2. It is much like a seesaw, where the balance is often tipped in favour of one more than the other. In terms of fertility, it's the TH cells that affect implantation of the embryo into the uterus wall. If TH1 is dominant, your body has more inflammation, which suppresses implantation. If TH2 is dominant, your body is less inflamed and the body allows the embryo to implant. Another way to look at it is to imagine your body as a castle, surrounded by a moat of water with a drawbridge, which is your immune system. Your body is constantly on the defence against potential attackers from outside the castle. During most of your menstrual cycle, the castle is prepared for attack and the drawbridge is up – TH1 is dominant. However, for four to five days of the month after ovulation, the drawbridge is down, your immune system is lowered and TH2 dominates, allowing implantation of the embryo into the uterus wall [62].

The immune system was once thought to be autonomous but new research has shown that its response is variable depending on the stress a person is under [63]. Stress can impact TH1 and TH2 ratio levels, depending upon what type of stress the person is experiencing and its severity. For example, trauma increases cytokine activity while bereavement reduces NK cell activity [63].

Research has confirmed acupuncture's ability to regulate the immune system, including NK cells [64]. Recent research conducted in South Korea has shown that the acupuncture channel network is contained within the lymphatic system (immune system), which allows acupuncture to effectively regulate immune factors [65]. Research into herbal medicine has shown that ginseng can regulate TH1 and TH2 levels thereby aiding an embryo implanting into the uterus lining [335] [336].

Self-Testing

You can do several tests yourself to see if there are other problems that can be addressed to improve your fertility. These tests can help you become more aware of yourself and your fertility. Take 10 minutes now to give them a try and see what you find:

- Sit down in a quiet place and start to meditate. A simple meditation technique is to focus on your breath entering and leaving your nose. Your mind needs something to focus upon and, as you need to breathe, you can put the two together. It helps bring your awareness back into your body, rather than being caught up in your thoughts. If you find it hard to meditate then your mind is overactive and possibly anxious. An overactive mind will consume important energy and blood that could otherwise be used for your fertility. Take time each day, starting off with five minutes, to practise meditation or mindfulness to quieten your mind and preserve your energy levels. If you try to meditate but fall asleep, then your body is tired and needs to recharge. Often our minds rule and dominate our bodies. The mind never gets tired and will wear the body out. This indicates a disconnect between mind and body. Try not to meditate when you're tired and sleep instead. There are many meditation apps that you can download onto your smartphone.

- If you have vivid dreams or wake up at around 4.30/5.30 a.m., then your mind is restless and anxious. The mind should settle deeply at night and not dream, in order for you to get deep good-quality sleep and wake feeling refreshed the next day. Waking early shows underlying anxiety, which is wearing the body out. Unfortunately, trying for a baby causes a lot of anxiety. This is where acupuncture can help to relax and calm the mind and emotions, improving sleep and boost the body's health.

- If you look in the mirror without make-up on and you look pale, then you may have a lack of blood, which can affect the thickness of the uterus lining and threaten a pregnancy in the early weeks. If you have dark circles under the eyes, then you may have a weak kidney, which can affect AMH levels and egg quality. If you suffer from dry skin, then you may have either a lack of blood (blood nourishes the skin), you don't drink enough fluids (you should drink 2 litres [½ gallon] a day) or you live in an area with hard water (use a water softener). If you're losing too much hair it can be a sign of a weak kidney or a lack of blood, or both. If you have a red face, then you have too much heat rising to the top of the body, caused by either excessive consumption of hot foods, such as chilli, and liquids, such as alcohol, or exposure to stress.

Western medicine is great for tests. Tests offer an invaluable insight into the inner workings of the body, which can give answers to infertility problems. However, what is often more important in today's world, are the causes of infertility and how to avoid them.

Chapter 4

The Causes of Infertility

The causes of infertility are often complex. In my experience, infertility is seldom a result of one problem; it's usually a combination of factors. Individually, these causes won't necessarily lead to infertility, but when combined together, they can. Without knowing, a lot of people are combining these causes together, thereby damaging their fertility and chances of having a baby. The best treatment strategy is to tackle all the various aspects together to form a strong combined treatment plan that will have the best result.

Both men and women can have reduced fertility. It is estimated that the cause is predominantly female in 38 per cent of couples and primarily male in 20 per cent, while 27 per cent both have abnormalities. For the remaining 15 per cent, no cause is found (in Western medicine) [13].

The common causes of infertility are numerous and include:

- age
- alcohol, smoking and illegal drugs
- environmental toxins, chemicals and pharmaceutical side effects
- excessive exercising
- free radicals
- genetics

- overworking
- poor diet
- stress and anxiety
- weight – both under- and overweight

Age

Age is an important factor in fertility. Both male and female fertility declines with age, but for women it often declines sooner than for men. However, often age is given too much importance in determining a woman's fertility. An older woman can still have children naturally, though they will be more in need of supplementation to aid their general health and egg quality.

As a general rule, most women's fertility reduces from the age of 35, but this isn't a cut-off point. You can still fall pregnant naturally after this age – it might just take a little more effort. For men, their fertility generally reduces from around the age of 45. Genetics play an important role in age-related infertility. A person who has inherited good genes can have children later in life, while another person may have inherited poor genes, which causes them to have fertility problems earlier in life.

As we age, we have fewer physical resources caused by living. Maintaining a good lifestyle and eating an optimised diet can help hold on to and replenish physical resources, such as energy, blood and lipids, allowing the body to be in a better position for natural conception.

Alcohol, Smoking and Illegal Drugs

Alcohol, smoking and even drugs (the illegal type) are commonplace today. Alcohol is by far the main drug of choice and the one that causes the most problems. Its use is seen as normal, and excessive use is often encouraged.

Alcohol

Alcohol is warm in Nature and drinking too much of it can cause excessive heat inside the body. This excessive heat is like the body being slowly cooked from the inside, damaging bodily fluids. In men this can cause reduced sperm motility, while in women it can lead to reduced cervical mucus, excessive menstrual bleeding, anaemia, reduced egg quality and reoccurring miscarriages, to name but a few.

In Western medicine alcohol affects the liver, whereas in Chinese medicine it affects the digestive and urinary systems. These systems become overloaded trying to detox alcohol from the body. With a weakened digestive system, the body becomes inefficient at processing food and normal fluids. This in turn leads to a weakness in the body with a lack of energy and blood, which reduces levels of leptin that reduces hormone regulation from the hypothalamus. This doesn't mean alcohol is completely bad, and while some people suggest not drinking any alcohol when trying for a baby, I recommend drinking just a little. Drinking two glasses of red wine a week can help blood, reduce stress and regulate hormones. But no more than two glasses (125ml/1.4 units per glass) a week! Red wine is preferred as it mimics the colour of blood. Other alcoholic drinks, such as spirits, are very hot in Nature and can create too much heat inside the body, which can affect bodily fluids and semen quality. Spirits should therefore be avoided. Beer and lager tend to be heavy on the digestive system, which can weaken it leading to a subsequent lack of energy and blood. I would therefore only recommend a couple of bottles of beer or lager a week.

Smoking

Smoking greatly affects both male and female fertility. In women, smoking affects the fallopian tubes causing blockages which can cause infertility and an increased risk of ectopic pregnancies [66]. Smoking also affects ovulation, the quality of the egg, fertilisation and the egg's ability to implant into the uterus wall [67]. Studies have shown that women who smoke took longer to fall pregnant naturally [68].

Smoking greatly damages male fertility. Men who smoke tend to drink alcohol as well. Male chronic users of nicotine and alcohol suffer from impotence, loss of libido, premature or delayed ejaculation and infertility. Clinical studies have confirmed that chronic consumption of alcohol and nicotine causes a decline in testosterone levels, a decreased sperm count and sperm maturation, leading to male infertility [69].

Nicotine affects the Leydig cell's production of testosterone, which is important in sperm production. Supplements such as passionflower (*passiflora incarnata linneaus*) can help reduce alcohol and nicotine's harmful effects upon male fertility [69]. However, it's best not to smoke at all when trying for a baby.

Illegal drugs

Illegal drugs, especially stimulants such as cocaine, crack and MDMA, create highs that greatly consume the body's deep reserves of energy. A reduction in these reserves can reduce the quality of the sperm and egg. Research has shown illegal drugs such THC, cocaine, crack and MDMA damage male fertility [70] [71] [72]. New research has shown that men who smoke cannabis for six months or more have altered DNA in their sperm [73].

Chemicals

We've finally reached the point at which our bodies are unable to evolve as quickly as our modern lives. Modern living started at the point of the Industrial Revolution. Initially, it brought prosperity and quicker ways of manufacturing and moving people and products from place to place. Eventually living standards improved, people's lives prospered and life expectancy increased. The point at which this peaked and the slow decline in fertility started was around the 1930s, during the Second World War.

It was during the 1940s that modern agricultural practices were established with the use of pesticides to kill off insects that would eat and damage crops, and herbicides to kill off weeds. These were introduced at a time when people could still remember the rationing of foods in Europe during the Second World War and they were therefore seen as necessary to feed the population. Throughout most of the 1950s, consumers and most policymakers were not concerned about the potential health risks of using pesticides. Food was cheaper because of these new chemicals and there were no documented cases of people dying or being seriously hurt by their use. It was around this time that male sperm concentrations started to decline [41].

As technology advanced, many chemicals were created to enhance our lives by killing bacteria to keep our living and working areas clean. Others were created to help clothe us, such as in the manufacturing of the synthetic polymers nylon and polyester. Chemicals were used in the farming of animals. Even more chemicals were created for healthcare, beauty and hygiene. Suddenly chemicals that don't exist in Nature were bombarding people's bodies. Our bodies come from Nature; they are not man-made and struggle to coexist with man-made chemicals. In this short space in our history, we have not evolved to live in harmony with such chemicals. This has led to the rise in ill health, infertility and other diseases such as cancer [74].

Although environmental chemicals have weak hormonal effects, they have the ability to interact with more than one. We are not exposed to one toxicant at a time, but rather, to hundreds if not thousands of man-made chemicals present in our environment. Collectively, they can be hazardous to human reproductive health [75].

Hormones in food

Foods derived from animals are an important source of nutrition and vitamins. Methods of production vary globally and include the use of hormones in cattle to increase growth and lean tissue with reduced fat. The hormonal compounds are naturally occurring in animals or are synthetically produced man-made chemicals that have an effect upon oestrogen and progesterone hormone activity. The use of synthetic hormones is still permitted in North American countries but is no longer allowed in Europe, which also prohibits the importation of meat and its products derived from hormone-treated cattle as it may induce free-radical damage of DNA [338]. Foods in North American countries are some of the most altered in the world.

The accumulation of endocrine-disrupting man-made chemicals (xenobiotics) in food sources, such as fish and animal meat, exposes people to increased concentrations of these compounds, which can have an effect upon both male and female fertility. Products from animal sources, such as cow's milk can also be a source of exposure to exogenous oestrogens [75].

Contaminated food and water may contain environmental pollutants, such as pesticide residues and heavy metals, in addition to processing aids and anabolic steroids used in food production, which disrupt normal hormone regulation. Most people have traceable amounts of these substances in their blood or urine [76]. Studies have shown how man-made hormones are causing infertility conditions such as premature ovarian failure, polycystic ovary syndrome (PCOS) and endometriosis [76].

Pesticides

Dichlorodiphenyltrichloroethane (DDT) does not occur naturally in the environment; it's a man-made chemical. Large amounts of DDT were released into the air and on soil or water when it was sprayed on crops and forests to kill insects. Organochlorine compounds, such as DDT, dichlorodiphenyldichloroethylene (DDE), and dichlorodiphenyldichloroethane (DDD), last in the soil for a very long time, potentially for hundreds of years [77]. Many studies have been conducted to determine the concentration of environmental contaminants, especially organochlorine compounds. Both DDT and DDE have been shown to reduce levels of oestrogens and progesterone leading to infertility and early pregnancy loss [78]. DDT was banned in the USA in 1972, but still lives on in our environment. Glyphosate is the world's most widely used herbicide. Research has linked an increased use of glyphosate with a reduced fertility [348] [349], an increase prevalence of attention deficit hyperactivity disorder (ADHD) in people [347] and an increase prevalence of autism [350] [351] [352] [353]. Other pesticides have been linked to an increase rate of children developing autism [340].

Hormones in water

In France, studies have identified numerous compounds in surface water (before treatment), including acetaminophen (paracetamol – tylenol), salicylic acid, analgesics, psychotropic drugs, antibiotics and beta blockers, as well as natural hormones (oestrogens, progesterone and androgens) and synthetic progesterone [79]. These compounds come from farming, the public (the contraceptive pill) and hospitals. The number of pharmaceuticals and hormones and their presence in the final waters indicate that most treatments fail in their total elimination [79]. Recent research found 11 pharmaceuticals in drinking waters from Germany, the UK, Italy, Canada and the USA [79]. The levels of hormones present are small, yet in conjunction with hormones in meat and beverages, as well as cosmetics and man-made products, their levels increase and can affect fertility in both men and women.

Another problem with disinfected drinking water is the by-products found in virtually all chlorinated water supplies. Research conducted in California found that women who drank more than five glasses of cold tap water a day, if it contained more than 75 micrograms per litre of total trihalomethanes (THMs), had an increase in miscarriage rates in their first trimester [80]. THM levels in tap water can also delay time to pregnancy [81].

Hormones in cosmetics

Man-made chemicals are commonly used in cosmetics too. Unlike soaps or shampoos, which are rinsed off, other cosmetics remain on the body for considerably longer. These man-made chemicals, such as parabens (in most make-up, moisturisers, haircare products and shaving products), antiperspirant aluminium salts, cyclosiloxanes (silicones, in combination or alone in personal care products and as carriers, lubricants and solvents), triclosan (found in antibacterial soaps and body washes, toothpastes and some cosmetics), ultraviolet (UV) screens and phthalates, have an oestrogenic potency and react like oestrogens, which can disrupt the normal balance of hormones in both men and women [82].

Phthalates and parabens are found in nail polish, cosmetics, lotions and in perfumes [83]. Women who use four or more personal care products (perfume, deodorant, lipstick, nail polish and hand/face cream, for example) have more than four times higher concentrations of phthalates than in women using only two or three products [84]. Pregnant mothers exposed to phthalates have an increased risk of their children developing autism [339] [340] [341].

Octamethylcyclotetrasiloxane (D4) is a colourless viscous liquid that is widely used in cosmetics. Research over the past four decades demonstrates the toxicity of D4 and its ability to interfere with female reproduction [82].

Naturally-occurring oestrogens (phytoestrogens) from plants are widely used in cosmetics too. Phytoestrogens are added to cosmetics in the form of anthraquinones present in aloe vera and in breast-enhancing creams in the form of 8-prenylnaringenin ('push-up') and miroestrol/deoxymiroestrol (pueraria creams). Many of these compounds are not readily metabolised and, due to their lipophilic properties, they can accumulate over time in fatty tissues of the body

[82]. They can then be released and, in conjunction with other oestrogen-type chemicals, cause hormonal imbalances and infertility.

Hormones in food packaging

Bisphenol A (BPA) was first synthesised in 1891, as a synthetic oestrogen. BPAs can cross the placenta – studies have found concentrations in both mother and foetus [85]. Exposure of the foetus to BPA can increase the risk of autism [340]. Tins in which foods are preserved are often lined with BPAs as are some coffee takeaway cups (see 'Know your plastics' on page 143).

Recent studies have concluded that plastic packaging is an important source of endocrine disruptors in the average human diet. Repeated exposure of food-contact materials to UV light, heat and acidic/alkaline contents may cause the polymers contained within the packaging to break down into monomers as phthalates and BPA, which then leach into food and beverages that are then consumed [76].

There is chronic intake of endocrine disruptors even from bottled water. Some of these endocrine disruptors are being replaced by other equally bad substances: many 'BPA-free' water containers contain bisphenol S (BPS) instead, which also exerts both genomic and non-genomic endocrine-disruptive effects upon the body [76].

Aniline

Aniline is used in meat production, cigarettes, pesticides, pharmaceuticals (acetaminophen - paracetamol - tylenol) colourants used in food, cosmetics and textiles [88]. If your mother, or your partner's mother, took paracetamol during pregnancy, you are both more likely to have reduced fertility [89] [90]. Paracetamol use has been shown in research to affect male fertility by delaying time to pregnancy and can prevent a woman from ovulating [88] [91].

Household hormones

Environmental hormones include numerous synthetic substances used as industrial lubricants and solvents and their by-products, for example PCBs and polybrominated diphenyl ethers (PBDEs, used as a flame retardant). PBDEs have been shown to affect male sperm quality [92]. Flame-retardant chemicals such as organophosphate (OP) compounds, have replaced PBDEs in recent years. OP compounds have been found in house dust, which is then digested by the occupants causing an increase in prolactin levels leading to an irregular menstrual cycle in women and a decrease in semen quality in men [93].

Alkylphenol ethoxylates (APEs)

APEs are detergents, emulsifiers and wetting agents used in paints, household products, toiletries, pesticides and many other industrial and agricultural products. Excessive exposure to APEs has been shown to affect male reproductive development [94].

Polychlorinated biphenyls (PCBs)

Polychlorinated biphenyls (PCBs) are found in meat, fish, poultry and in the tissues of humans. PCBs have been linked to male infertility and early puberty in girls [87]. PCBs can alter thyroid hormone activity [86], which is important in the luteal phase (second half) of the menstrual cycle. PCBs have been detected in the seminal fluid of infertile men, causing them to have lower ejaculate volume, sperm count, progressive motility, normal morphology and fertilising ability [87].

Polyfluorinated chemicals (PFCs)

PFCs are also known as perfluorinated chemicals, perfluorochemicals, perfluoroalkyls, perfluorinated alkyl acids, polyfluorinated chemicals, polyfluorinated compounds and polyfluoroalkyl substances. In recent years, PFCs have increasingly been investigated for their potential harm to humans.

PFCs are a large group of manufactured compounds that are widely used to make everyday products designed to repel soil, grease and water, including: carpet and furniture treatments; food wraps; sprays for leather, shoes and other clothing; paints and cleaning products; and even in products like shampoo and floor wax. PFCs may be used to keep food from sticking to cookware (non-stick frying pans, i.e. Du Pont's Telfon pans), to make sofas and carpets resistant to stains, to make clothes and mattresses more waterproof and may also be used in some food packaging (such as fast food containers or microwave popcorn bags), as well as in some firefighting materials [95].

The most well-known PFCs are perfluorooctane sulfonic acid (PFOS), perfluorooctanoic acid (PFOA) and their derivatives belonging to the group of perfluoroalkylated substances. PFCs are very persistent in the environment and some of them have been discovered as global pollutants of air, water, soil and wildlife. Bioaccumulation occurs in humans and everybody in our society has traces of these PFCs in their blood and internal organs such as the liver, kidneys, spleen, gall bladder and testes [95]. Some of these PFCs, such as PFOS and PFOA, are potential developmental toxicants and are suspected endocrine disruptors with effects on sex hormone levels resulting in lower testosterone levels and higher oestradiol levels [95]. Most westernised countries have now banned their use. However, hundreds of related chemicals are not regulated and could potentially affect fertility hormone levels.

The major human exposure to PFCs is most likely from surfactants used for impregnation of consumer goods, such as textiles, footwear, furniture and carpets, which then release PFCs to the indoor air and contaminate indoor dust, which is then inhaled by people. Babies and toddlers may be more exposed to house dust while playing on the floor and will then collect these contaminated dusts on their fingers and put them in their mouth and ingest them. Relative to body weight children have a 5–10 times larger intake of indoor PFCs than adults [95].

Two recent studies suggest that PFCs may reduce human fertility. In Danish women, higher PFOS and PFOA levels were associated with a longer time to pregnancy and irregular menstrual cycles [95]. Young Danish men with high combined PFOS and PFOA levels had half the number of normal sperm compared to men with lower levels [96]. This lower sperm count could be due to the effects of polyfluorinated substances on Leydig cells. Leydig cells, which produce testosterone in men, are commonly enlarged (hyperplasia) amongst infertile men, leading to lower testosterone levels and high oestrogen levels [95].

International awareness and concern is increasing. In 2000 the main producer, the 3M Company, voluntarily stopped the production of one of the chemicals (PFOS) and a ban of some fluorotelomers was introduced in Canada in 2006 [95]. In Europe, PFOS and its derivatives were banned in 2008, while in the USA they were banned in 2000 [95]. However, in China, PFOS levels have increased exponentially since 2003. Levels of PFOS in Shenyang, China in 2004 were approximately seven times higher than those found in the US general population at that time [97]. PFOS are only a small part of the problem. The family of PFCs consists of several hundred other unrestricted chemicals.

Fossil fuels

Other environmental pollutants include those from the burning of wood and secondary cigarette smoke. The burning of wood releases a number of pollutants including polychlorinated dibenzodiozins and dibenzofurans, polychlorinated biphenyls, particulate matter and polycyclic aromatic hydrocarbons (PAHs). Pregnant women exposed to PAHs are at greater risk of their baby developing intrauterine growth retardation (IUGR) or being born with a low birth weight [109]. Other research has shown that women with long-term exposure to smoke from either cigarettes or the burning of wood in their homes are more likely to have lower levels of anti-Müllerian hormone

(AMH) and reduced fertility [25]. Research has shown that breathing in second-hand cigarette smoke before conceiving can affect the baby's brain [98]. Other air pollutants, such as those from diesel car engines, have been linked to an increase rate of autism amongst children [340].

Oral contraceptive pill

Taking contraceptives is common amongst women today. They are often prescribed to teenage girls to alleviate menstrual pain, moderate their hormones and skin, and prevent unwanted pregnancies. Girls often continue without a break for over a decade until they meet someone and settle down, only to find they can't fall pregnant. Research has shown that women who had taken the combined pill took significantly longer to fall pregnant after coming off the pill [99]. The situation was worse for women who were over 35, obese or had irregular periods. In my clinic, I've found that women who've been taking contraceptives for over a decade find it hard to fall pregnant. The body is not a machine where a switch can be flicked to turn fertility back on or off, which is very much how Western medicine sees it.

Today, most oral contraceptive pills use a combination of hormones – oestrogens and progestins – hence their name: the combined pill. They work by suppressing follicle stimulating hormone (FSH) and luteinising hormone (LH) thereby preventing ovulation. They also thicken cervical mucus making it more difficult for the sperm to use it as a ladder to climb up and enter the uterus. Progestogen-only contraceptive pills (the mini pill or 'POP') make the cervical mucus too thick, thereby preventing the sperm from travelling up into the uterus and impregnating the egg. They also prevent the pituitary gland from sending out LH, which prevents ovulation and makes the uterus lining inhospitable.

Contraceptive skin implants are popular amongst younger women. In my experience, the use of these causes great hormonal imbalances, weight gain and emotional disturbances. The implant can also become dislodged and lost in the body. Menstrual cycles can take even longer to normalise once the implant has been removed from the body [99].

The future

Out of a chemical universe topping 80,000 substances, over 1000 have laboratory evidence of adverse effects, but only a small fraction have been studied in humans [100]. Only 40 chemicals that are widely distributed in the environment have been reported to have effects on reproduction or to have other hormonal-disrupting effects. However, this number must be considered incomplete, since literally tens-of-thousands of the man-made chemicals have yet to be evaluated for their effects upon male and female fertility.

Poor Diet

Our food, which has been tampered with since the 1940s, is now even more processed to make its shelf life longer and to make it look more appetising. Food is available in pre-packed plastics with chemicals added to it to make its shelf-life longer (as if there weren't enough already from the spraying of crops and processing). It's then made into a ready-made meal with added salt, sugar and preservatives, and then finally zapped in a microwave (see page 170) to take the last bit of goodness out of it, ready for us to eat.

We eat on the go, at our desks while stressed at work and late at night after a long day at the office, thus impairing digestion by not allowing the food to digest properly. This in turn affects our sleep and reduces our energy levels further, for us to wake and repeat. It only takes a few years of this cycle to weaken the body enough to damage fertility.

Weight

Weight is a known factor in health, but it can also affect fertility. Being either overweight or underweight can damage your fertility. If you're underweight (less than 22 per cent body fat), it can mean your oestrogen levels may be lower than normal, which can cause infertility. The body may also have some type of deficiency, such as energy and blood. This can lead to amenorrhoea (no period), anovulation (not ovulating), poor egg quality (chromosome abnormalities) and reoccurring miscarriages. Eating regularly and reducing exercise will help to recover body fat levels, improving the body's health and fertility. Having regular acupuncture will help with blood circulation and hormone regulation, and will aid the body's digestive system to produce more blood. Chinese herbs are very helpful in rebuilding deficiencies that have come about by not eating properly or from over-exercising.

Leptin

Women who diet and feel hungry are more likely to have low levels of LH and leptin. Leptin is a hormone that makes us feel satiated after eating. When energy reserves rise above a certain level, leptin levels increase to a threshold concentration signalling to the central nervous system (hypothalamus) that the body can now support reproduction [101] [102] [103]. Leptin also stimulates the pituitary gland to produce FSH and LH [102]. It's therefore not good to diet or fast when trying for a baby as this can cause irregular hormone levels. Leptin mainly exists in fatty tissues, which is one reason why women with less than 22 per cent body fat tend not to have adequate levels of leptin and develop an irregular menstrual cycle.

The hormone ghrelin, which is released by the stomach when we are hungry, also has the same effect on fertility hormone release by affecting the hypothalamus and the release of FSH and LH [104]. We should therefore be careful not to go hungry for too long or overeat as both can affect hormone regulation and fertility.

Overweight

A lot of women I see for fertility are concerned about their weight. Unfortunately being overweight can also interfere with fertility. Too much fat in the body increases levels of proteins that mediate implantation of the embryo to the uterus lining, called advanced glycation end products (AGEs) [1]. Fat contains oestrogens, which can affect levels of oestradiol in the body, causing infertility conditions such as endometriosis. Women who are overweight will tend to have higher levels of insulin too. Insulin reduces the levels of sex hormone-binding globulin (SHBG), causing more circulating testosterone in the body, which over feed the ovaries leading to multiple follicles, none of which mature (PCOS). Obesity may also be associated with a mild iron deficiency because of subclinical inflammation, increased hepcidin levels (a peptide hormone that regulates iron levels) and decreased iron absorption, leading to a pattern where infertility can form [105]. Women who are over-weight at the time of conceiving have a greater risk of their children developing autism [15].

If you think you are overweight, measure your waist–hip ratio. This is done by dividing your waist measurement by your hip measurement. Do not use body mass index (BMI) as this is out of date. If your waist–hip ratio is 0.8 or higher, then your fertility would benefit from some weight loss [106].

Excessive Exercising

Exercise, like everything else in life, is good only in moderation. Too little of it causes tiredness, stagnation, stress and ill health, whereas too much can weaken the body and damage fertility. Excessive exercising is perceived as a healthy endeavour in Western culture, but exercising, like all activities in life, requires energy and blood. Doing too much of it will spend the body's energy and blood reserves, leaving the body weakened. Research has shown that women who exercise too much have reduced fertility [107], while men that enter triathlons or lift weights every day, can have reduced sperm quality too.

Overworking

In a global economy, we now compete with others around the world for money and prosperity. This causes the companies that we work for to be more aggressive in their business dealings that make us work harder for longer, to drive up profits for their shareholders. It's a downward trend towards burnout, a burnout that greatly damages our health and fertility. This can be clearly seen in Japan, where people work 60–100 hours of overtime a month, leading to the highest use of IVF in the world [108]. Research has shown that working more than 40 hours a week damages fertility [54].

Most people I see in my clinic are mainly affected by overworking and long commutes to work. Working late with early starts is akin to burning the candle at both ends, which weakens the body.

Couples trying for an additional child tend to fall into this category of being overworked. Having children is life-changing and often results in a lack of sleep, excessive work for both women and men, and subsequent physical weakness. Secondary infertility, where a couple have demonstrated fertility but are struggling to fall pregnant again, can come as a surprise when their previous children may have been conceived easily.

Free Radicals

Our primary need to survive on this planet is to breathe in oxygen (O_2). The well-known by-product of breathing in oxygen is carbon dioxide (CO_2), while a lesser well-known by-product is reactive oxygen species (ROS). ROS are free radicals. A free radical is an unpaired electron. A certain amount of free radicals are needed for fertility, to help the uterus lining shed with each menstrual bleed and help with fertilisation and implantation. But too many can stress the body, at a cellular level. When the balance between free radicals and antioxidants is tipped towards an overabundance of free radicals, oxidative stress occurs. Breathing in air pollution ($PM_{2.5}$) can also cause oxidative stress [109]. Once the balance shifts, these highly reactive radicals can start a chain reaction, like dominoes. Their chief danger comes from the damage they can do when they react with important cellular components, such as DNA in the sperm head or the cell membrane of an egg. Cells may function poorly or die ('apoptosis'). To prevent free radical damage the body has a balancing system of antioxidants, such as melatonin, vitamins C and E, beta-carotene and selenium.

Antioxidants are molecules that can safely interact with free radicals and terminate the chain reaction before other molecules are damaged. The most potent antioxidant is melatonin. The body can only produce melatonin while sleeping at night-time. Sleeping in the daytime decreases melatonin production as sunlight reduces its release, unless the room is completely devoid of light [110]. The other antioxidants must be supplied from your diet. Older women tend to have low levels of antioxidants and high levels of free radicals [111]. This imbalance may be one reason for poor egg quality and an increase in birth defects.

High levels of oxidants can damage the egg after its release from the ovary, the embryo and, most importantly, sperm, which are highly sensitive to oxidative stress [112]. Once damaged by excessive free radicals, the damage cannot be reversed. Fluid around the follicles contains high levels of antioxidants, which protect eggs and sperm from damage caused by too many free radicals. Women with low levels of free radicals have a greater rate of their eggs becoming blastocysts [113].

Inflammation or infection can increase levels of free radicals produced by the male's immune system via high levels of white blood cells (known as 'leukocytospermia') present in the semen. There are various markers that are used to test levels of oxidative stress, for example total antioxidant capacity (TAC), which is measured together with ROS to determine male fertility. A level of TAC-ROS below 30 is considered poor. Men who smoke have a low TAC-ROS score. In addition there is TAC plus lipoperoxidation (LPO), which is used to measure oxidative stress in women. Levels of LPO and TAC are significantly lower in women who do not become pregnant than in those who do.

An increase in levels of free radicals initiates an inflammatory response via cytokines along the lymphatic system. Modern research has shown the chain reaction of free radicals follows paths that are almost identical to acupuncture channels [114]. This ties in with other research that has found the acupuncture channels within the lymphatic system [115]. It may therefore be possible for acupuncture to act like an antioxidant and stop the chain reaction caused by too many free radicals.

Stress and Anxiety

As technology has grown with the promise of making our lives easier, we have surrounded ourselves with computers and gadgets, often becoming addicted to them. Technology may well have made our lives easier in some ways, but a negative side effect has made us less able to switch off our minds, which makes us stressed and anxious. We are constantly plugged in, almost permanently wired up to receive information, whether it's from smartphones, tablets, multiple televisions with hundreds of channels, the radio, the Internet, etc. We are constantly being bombarded with massive amounts of information on a daily basis.

This amount of data needs to be processed by our minds all the time. It's organised, filed away and called upon to talk about with other people, friends or even strangers over the airwaves and the Internet. Social media sites are terrible for this. They offer small amounts of data and cookies, which act like crack for the mind, constantly feeding it until the mind becomes bloated and obese with information and is unable to be tamed, causing a restless mind, anxiety, stress and sleeping problems.

Processing vast amounts of information on a daily basis is very energy-dependent and taxing. We haven't evolved quickly enough like our modern machines to be so energy efficient, which makes us tired, and that damages fertility.

People have forgotten how to relax. I notice this a lot when people get off my couch after having acupuncture treatment and can't believe how relaxed they feel; it's something they seldom feel any more.

Genetics

Genetics play an important role in fertility. Genetics mean that we have a probable predisposition to travel a certain fertility path. However, we can change the path if we live by the laws of Nature and look after our health by using the information contained within this book and listen to our bodies.

I'm already seeing women in my clinic whose mothers had fertility problems and were given fertility drugs. They are finding their own fertility is a problem but at a much younger age. This is something I call 'inherited premature infertility' (IPI). Some women who are in their early thirties have the fertility of a 40-year-old. This is due to their constitution. Our constitution – how healthy we are and therefore how good our fertility can be – is inherited from our parents through our genes. For example, if your mother had fertility issues, then you are more likely to have the same issues or if your mother suffered from a blood deficiency, then you may also have a lack of blood. Likewise, on the other hand, if your mother had children later in life, then you may also be able to.

Part Two

Chinese Medicine and Fertility

From a Chinese medical viewpoint, fertility is more than just eggs and the uterus lining they burrow into. Chinese medicine zooms out to look at the whole person. All aspects of a woman and man are important for their fertility – not just the nuts and bolts of their reproductive systems. For example, emotions, energy levels, weight, diet, exercise, sleep, blood, cold and heat all have an effect upon the body and need to be balanced to enhance fertility. These are things that you can easily balance yourself by taking on the advice contained within this book.

Chapter 5

The Fundamentals of Chinese Medicine

Firstly, let me give you some background theory about Chinese medicine. Chinese medicine sees everything in duality: heaven–earth, yin–yang, sun–moon, male–female, sperm–egg, etc. There must be balance between these elements of duality in order to have good health and fertility.

Yin and yang

Yin and yang is the most important concept in Chinese medicine. Most people have heard of yin and yang but perhaps don't know how they relate to fertility. Women are predominantly yin, while men are predominantly yang. Oestrogens are yin while testosterone is yang. Follicle stimulating hormone (FSH) is yin while luteinising hormone (LH) is yang and so on. Yin and yang should be in balance. When they fall out of balance, dis-ease occurs. If you have too much yang then you will have too much heat, which can cause poor sperm motility and threaten a pregnancy. If you have a deficiency of yin, you can have low levels of cervical mucus and poor egg and sperm quality. Everything can be broken down into either yin or yang (see table 5 on page 80–81).

Yin and yang can also change into each other. This is illustrated by the famous yin and yang symbol with the small circle in each part;

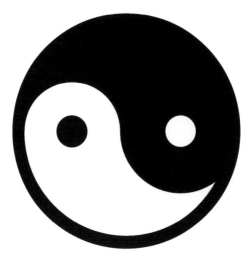

Figure 4. Yin and yang symbol

the black dot in the white and the white dot in the black (see above). The same principle can be applied to fertility hormones. When there is too much testosterone in a woman – a male/yang hormone – it increases male characteristics such as facial hair and can cause infertility. When there is too much oestrogen in a man, it creates female characteristics, such as enlarged breasts, and can reduce fertility.

Yin and yang are rooted in Nature. They come from observing the world around us. If we fight against the laws of Nature, our health suffers and we develop infertility. For example, night-time is the time of yin. This is when we should be at our most inactive and should rest and sleep. If we stay up late and continue to work long hours into the night, it will make us more deficient, which will damage yin and our fertility [116].

You can see by looking at the table 6 below how problems with yin or yang can be translated into fertility. For example, a deficiency of yin can manifest as:

- a lack of blood (anaemia)
- an irregular follicular phase
- high FSH levels

- little or no cervical mucus
- low levels of oestrogens
- problems with either the sperm or the egg
- reoccurring miscarriages

A deficiency of yang can manifest as:

- a poor LH surge
- low progesterone levels
- low testosterone levels
- problems with the rupturing of the follicle and release of the egg
- problems with the sperm penetrating the egg
- the embryo unable to burrow into the uterus wall

Acupuncture is good at balancing these forces within the body, which aids general health and fertility. However, acupuncture cannot give you more yin or yang, energy or blood. What it can do is help the body create them itself. Chinese herbs can give the body what it needs, i.e. more energy (qi), blood, yin or yang. This is why Chinese herbs are considered stronger than acupuncture and are a more popular form of treatment in China.

Yin	Yang
General	
Female	Male
Moon	Sun
Water	Fire
Earth	Heaven
Night	Day
Midnight	Midday
Cold	Hot
Passive	Active
Below	Above

Fertility	
Antioxidants	Free radicals
Blood	Energy (qi)
Cervical mucus	Semen
Egg	Sperm
Essential fatty acids	Protein
Follicular phase	Luteal phase
FSH	LH
Implantation	Embryo transportation
Oestrogens	Progesterone
Ovulation	Fertilisation
Oxytocin	Testosterone
Pregnancy	Labour
Sedentary	Exercise
Seminal fluid	Sperm
Sperm head	Sperm tail
Sperm morphology	Sperm motility
TH2	TH1

Table 5. A comparison of yin and yang in fertility

Qi

Qi (pronounced 'chee') is the same as energy. However, in East Asia, energy has more functions than just giving us oomph and power [117]. It holds our organs in place and keeps them up so they don't prolapse, including the embryo or foetus. It also protects the body from viruses and bacteria by maintaining the immune system. It keeps the body warm, including the uterus, thereby making it a suitable environment for your baby to grow. For these reasons, qi is yang in Nature.

Western medicine can measure a person's energy expenditure and energy intake, but it cannot measure their current energy level. Chinese medicine can measure the current energy level of a person through pulse diagnosis [118].

Energy levels decrease with age. You may see young people walking around in the cold wearing fewer clothes than others. This is because as they are young, they have more energy, which aids in keeping them warm (yang). In the elderly, they are often cold and need to heat their homes more than younger people, as they have less energy (yang), as they have spent it through living.

To help you understand how energy works and how it can affect your health and fertility, I will use a simple analogy: energy is like money. We convert our energy through work into money, which we use to buy food to give us energy. We also spend energy when we exercise excessively, overwork and don't sleep enough. Most people's energetic outgoings are greater than their energetic income, which weakens the body and damages fertility. They are spending more than they receive. Over time, with career promotions, socialising and living life to the full, this can make the body physically weak, leaving a deficit in their fertility account (see Figure 5 below). This can reduce levels of leptin which affect normal hormone release from the hypothalamus. It's therefore important to manage and budget energy expenditure to improve your fertility. This comes from being more aware of your energy levels and your body's needs. It won't take long for you to become more aware of your energy and where you are spending it. With more awareness comes greater fertility!

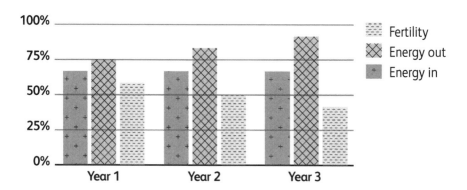

Figure 5. An estimate of energy intake and expenditure affecting fertility over time

When asked, most people will say their energy levels are good, only for me to check their pulse and find that it's weak. This is because most people have their awareness plugged into their mind. We are more than our minds; we are the awareness that sits behind the mind. If you can unplug your awareness from your mind and plug it into your body, most people will find their body is weak and wants to rest. You can unplug your awareness from your mind through activities such as meditation, yoga and mindfulness.

As a potential parent, it's likely that you are happy to sacrifice a part of your health for your baby, but unfortunately your body doesn't work like this. It's a survival organism that will only support the baby if you, the mother, have enough energy after your daily needs have been met. Energy is finite – there's only so much you have. If you spend too much of your energy working, commuting, socialising, exercising or using technology such as social media, you will have less energy and fewer resources left over for your fertility (see Figure 6 below).

To improve your fertility, you need to do less and conserve resources to support and grow your baby. Doing less is difficult for most people as our minds tell us we need to work hard to get what we want or finish off those things on our 'to-do list' before we can allow ourselves to relax. In terms of fertility, it's the opposite: doing less can actually improve your fertility. Try to start listening to your body rather than your mind as it's your body that will have your baby, not your mind!

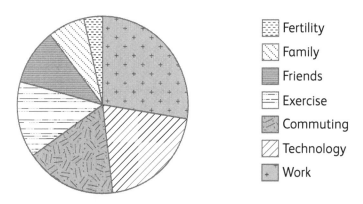

Figure 6. An estimate of energy expenditure in a typical person

Blood

Blood is the same in Chinese medicine as it is in Western medicine. If you're anaemic in Western medicine, you'll be lacking in blood in Chinese medicine. However, there are two distinct differences:

1. Chinese medicine will diagnose you as lacking in blood a lot sooner than Western medicine. This is because the Western medical range of what is a good amount of blood is narrow and relates to illnesses such as anaemia. The range in Chinese medicine is a lot broader, allowing practitioners to identify a lack of blood sooner and treat it in order to optimise a person's health and fertility long before it's allowed to become a problem.

2. In Chinese medicine, overdoing it can reduce levels of blood in the body. Just as when you do too much and you feel tired and have a lack of energy, you also can have a lack of blood. Levels of blood can fluctuate like energy levels and affect your fertility. A good example of this is during a woman's menstrual cycle, when the blood loss can make a lot of women feel tired, drained and dizzy.

Blood does more than just move oxygen around the body; it carries your fertility hormones and immune system, it's needed to thicken the uterus lining and grow the placenta as well as helping your baby to grow. Blood goes hand-in-hand with energy. Where energy goes, blood goes. When we are tired we often think we have a lack of energy, but we can also have a lack of blood [105]. This is why taking an iron supplement, which increases the amount of red blood cells (haemoglobin) in the body, can make us feel less tired.

The body is very much in the now and will react to the environment it is put in. Working or commuting long hours will deplete energy and blood as people are spending more of their body's resources than they are receiving through food and sleep. The body simply reacts to this as it thinks it needs to spend these resources. If your job or commute is stressful, then even more of your body's resources are consumed, leaving you more energy- and blood-deficient, worsening your fertility.

Your body doesn't hear that your job isn't as important as having a baby; it just sees what's going out of your energy account and what's left over for your fertility. Over a few years, this constant spending of more energy and blood than you are putting in can affect sperm and egg quality, the thickness of the uterus lining and even hormone levels such as FSH (see Figure 5, page 82). Take a look at your energy expenditure and try to see where you can make savings.

A light menstrual flow that never becomes heavy is convenient for most women as it is less hassle, but in Chinese medicine it actually shows a lack of blood and poor fertility. A good period flow should last between five and seven days and be heavy for the first 3–5 days, then reduce to medium, then light. Being dizzy during your period can be a sign of a deficiency of blood.

As blood is a liquid the surrounding temperature affects its flow. When the body is cold, blood doesn't flow around the body as well as it should do. Exposure to cold can affect the distribution of fertility hormones [11]. It's therefore important to keep your body warm and wear enough clothing and have warm foods and fluids to ensure that your blood flows better and your fertility hormones are well-regulated.

Jing

Jing translates into English as 'essence' [342]. Essence is a more concentrated form of yin. It's like concentrated moisturising cream but in a fluid form that the body uses. It's related to egg and sperm quality. Any chromosome abnormalities of the egg, poor egg reserves or morphology (physical structure) issues with the sperm show a deficiency of jing. Jing is housed in the kidneys. We are born with a set amount of it that we inherit from our parents and which we in turn pass on to our children.

If your jing is deficient then the body is exhausted, which may cause problems conceiving and can be a factor in reoccurring miscarriages. A poor diet, genetics or working long hours over many years can deplete jing levels.

Understanding what imbalance you have can help you focus on what you need to change in order to improve your health and have a baby naturally. Next, we'll look at the different types of imbalances within Chinese medicine and how you can treat them.

Chapter 6

Finding Your Chinese Medicine Diagnosis

In this chapter, I'll explain each of the patterns that exist in Chinese medicine. Understanding which category you fall into is important as it allows you to understand how one problem will affect the whole body, including your fertility, and what you can do about it. By joining up the dots and seeing the bigger picture, you can empower yourself to improve your fertility and your chances of having a baby naturally.

Once you've read through the different patterns, you may find that you fit into one or more types. This is because the majority of people don't fall into just one pattern, but are a mix of patterns, for example blood deficient with blood stasis, kidney yang deficiency with some liver qi stagnation and spleen qi deficiency. The trick is to determine which pattern is the dominant type and focus on fixing that first, then once another pattern becomes dominant, focus on that.

Qi Deficiency

In Chinese medicine there are many different types of energy and a lack of energy can do more than just make you feel tired.

Symptoms

Symptoms of a qi deficiency include:

- absence of a menstrual period (amenorrhoea)
- addiction to coffee
- dizziness
- heavy periods (menorrhagia)
- irregular menstrual cycles
- loose bowels
- painful periods (dysmenorrhoea)

- poor appetite
- prolapsed uterus
- reoccurring colds
- shortness of breath
- sweating in the day time
- tense muscles
- tired after exercising
- weak voice

Testing

There are various ways to test your energy levels, from your pulse or after practising certain activities. For example, if you meditate but fall asleep then you are tired, or if you feel tired after exercising then you have weak energy levels. Generally, however, Chinese medicine is symptom-driven, so if you have three or more of the above symptoms, you may be deficient in qi.

Causes

Energy can be depleted in many ways: working or exercising too much, not eating enough, dieting, a lack of sleep, anxiety, stress, etc. Emotional stress can deplete qi (energy) making you feel tired and down. This is known as the resistance phase in Western medicine, where the increase in circulating glucocorticoid hormones increases energy demands. Unfortunately, trying for a baby is very emotional and this in itself can deplete qi, which can reduce levels of leptin and cause irregular hormone levels.

Qi comes from the food and fluids we eat and from the air we breathe. Therefore, the quality of what we eat and the air we breathe is important in maintaining good energy levels. In Chinese medicine qi is greatly attributed to the spleen. Foods that damage the spleen's function, such as excessive dairy and gluten, can reduce a person's energy levels. Eating foods that are processed or are poor quality, such as prepared microwave meals, can also affect energy levels.

Eating like this for a long period of time can create a substantial lack of energy (see Figure 5, page 82), which can then damage fertility. Coffee is a powerful yang-moving stimulant, hence why a lot of people who are lacking in energy are addicted to it.

Risks

The health risks of having a deficiency of qi include:

- ectopic pregnancies
- implantation failure
- reoccurring miscarriage
- unexplained infertility

Treatment

Treatment strategies to improve energy levels include optimising all aspects of life – from diet, through to sleep and the clothes you wear – together in a programme to reduce energy expenditure and build up qi levels.

Treatment checklist ☑

- ☐ Avoid eating takeaways or microwave meals.
- ☐ Don't eat too late (after 7 p.m.).
- ☐ Don't work more than 40 hours a week.
- ☐ Eat high-quality, organic fruits and vegetables.
- ☐ Eat only organic, fresh meat (not from frozen).
- ☐ Exercise three times a week, but no more.
- ☐ Have weekly acupuncture treatment and take Chinese herbs such as ginseng.
- ☐ If stress is chronic, have counselling.
- ☐ Practise qi gong exercises.
- ☐ Reduce your consumption of coffee, sugar, gluten and dairy.
- ☐ Reduce your exposure to stress or emotional upset by distracting yourself with nice, fun things.
- ☐ Sleep before 10 p.m.

Blood Deficiency (Anaemia)

Within Western medicine understanding, a lack of blood is termed a lack of red blood cells (haemoglobin). This condition is very common, especially in women because they lose blood every month through their menstrual cycle.

Symptoms

Symptoms of a blood deficiency in Chinese medicine are common and most women will have some of the following:

- absence of a menstrual period (amenorrhoea)
- absence of ovulation (anovulation)
- addiction to coffee
- anxiety
- cold hands and feet
- cravings for sugar

- depression
- dizziness
- dreams
- dry skin
- high FSH levels
- insomnia
- irregular hormones
- irritability
- late periods
- light menstrual bleed
- numbness or tingling in the hands or feet
- pale complexion
- pale fingernails
- pale lips
- polycystic ovary syndrome (PCOS)
- poor memory
- scanty periods
- tiredness
- thin uterus lining

Testing

A lack of haemoglobin is often due to a lack of iron. There are six classifications of an iron deficiency in Western medicine, with the last being the most severe:

1. Iron deficiency.
2. Functional iron deficiency.
3. Iron deficiency anaemia.
4. Iron-refractory iron deficiency anaemia (IRIDA).
5. Anaemia of chronic diseases.
6. Iron deficiency and anaemia of chronic diseases [119].

Iron deficiency anaemia often remains undiagnosed and untreated [119]. Western medical doctors tend to only give iron support when iron levels are in the range of iron deficiency anaemia (category 3) [119]. By this time, damage has been done to your health and fertility. Most people are unaware that they are anaemic [120]. A blood deficiency is picked up earlier in Chinese medicine and can be treated sooner, thereby preventing any damage to fertility.

Causes

There are three organs involved in blood within Chinese medicine: the spleen, kidney and liver. The spleen turns foods and fluids we consume into energy and blood. The kidneys house the yin and jing, which go towards blood production. The liver moves and stores the blood.

The flavour associated with the spleen is sweet. Sweet foods help to generate blood. When people crave sugar, they are often deficient in blood. In Western medicine, this is similar. Blood sugar levels affect energy levels. People with low blood sugar levels (hypoglycaemia) will often be very tired and pale, which are symptoms of a blood deficiency in Chinese medicine.

The liver and the brain require a constant supply of blood sugar. Emotional stress affects the liver and can increase the need for blood sugar, making the person feel weak. Excessive mental activity, such as anxiety and prolonged stressful situations, also uses a lot of blood sugar, which again will make a person feel weak and their fertility will be damaged by having lower levels of leptin, which causes irregular levels of fertility hormones from the hypothalamus.

Overworking, sleeping late or going for long periods of sleep deprivation, poor diet, dieting, excessive exercising or blood loss from surgery, injuries or from heavy menstrual bleeds can all lead to a deficiency of blood. Drugs such as glucocorticoids, salicylates, nonsteroidal anti-inflammatory drugs (NSAIDs) and proton-pump inhibitors can reduce levels of iron in the body, which can affect levels of blood [105].

Risks

Blood plays a vital role in the regulation of fertility hormones and the immune system. It also nourishes the uterus lining ready for implantation and makes up a large part of the placenta. Blood works in conjunction with qi, which moves the blood and helps to transport it to all areas of the body where it is needed. The risks of having a deficiency of blood include:

- absence of a menstrual period (amenorrhoea)
- endometriosis
- implantation failure
- irregular menstrual cycles
- PCOS
- reoccurring miscarriage
- unexplained infertility

Treatment

Instead of eating sugary foods, which only gives a short burst of energy, eat foods with more protein and iron, as these will build long-lasting supplies of blood. Coffee moves blood, but the downside of this is that coffee can damage blood and fertility. Have a ginseng drink instead of coffee. Take an iron supplement too (see page 191).

Treatment checklist ☑

- ☐ Avoid refined sugar and coffee.
- ☐ Do not go for long periods with sleep deprivation.
- ☐ Don't exercise when having your menstrual bleed.
- ☐ Don't work more than 40 hours a week.
- ☐ Eat protein and iron rich foods.
- ☐ Have weekly acupuncture treatment and take Chinese herbs daily.
- ☐ Reduce your energy expenditure and exercise less.
- ☐ Sleep before 10 p.m.
- ☐ Take iron supplements (20mg) on top of your prenatal supplement.

Qi Stagnation

Qi (energy) stagnation is energy that doesn't move properly.

Symptoms

A stagnation of qi can cause the following symptoms:

- absence of a menstrual period (amenorrhoea)
- breast lumps
- breast tenderness
- bruise easily
- cysts
- depression
- haemorrhoids
- irregular menstrual cycles
- irritability
- mood swings
- muscle tension
- pain
- painful periods (dysmenorrhoea)
- premenstrual syndrome (PMS)
- repeated sighing
- seasonal affective disorder (SAD)

Testing

The way to test for qi stagnation is to look at the above symptoms and see if you have three or more of them. If so, then it's possible you may have a stagnation of qi.

Causes

A poor diet or excessive exercising or not exercising enough can cause a stagnation of energy. Emotional imbalances, such as frustration, resentment or worry, can also lead to a stagnation of qi. When qi is stagnated, blood will also become stagnated, as where energy goes, blood goes.

During the winter months we will often feel the effects of qi stagnation, as qi tends to stagnate easily when it's cold. It's also darker outside, which negatively affects our mood, and affects our energy flow. In these months, it helps our health if we slow down, do less and sleep and eat more, as if semi-hibernating in preparation for the more active summer months ahead. This helps to conserve important qi, blood and yin levels for later use for your fertility.

Risks

A stagnation of qi can cause:

- irregular menstrual cycles
- unexplained infertility

Treatment

The liver is the most affected organ when there is a stagnation of qi, as the liver is responsible for the regulation of qi in the body. Trying to conceive for a long time and not falling pregnant or having reoccurring miscarriages will cause emotional upset that can lead to a stagnation of qi. In such cases talking about your emotions with your partner, friends, relatives or a professional counsellor will help to resolve them and allow qi to flow better, thereby improving your fertility.

Treatment checklist ☑

- ☐ Don't eat foods that will bloat you, such as gluten and junk food.
- ☐ Exercise three to four times a week.
- ☐ Have weekly acupuncture treatment.
- ☐ Make sure you wear enough clothes to keep your body warm.
- ☐ Meditate or practise mindfulness.
- ☐ Practise yoga or t'ai chi regularly.
- ☐ Reduce your exposure to the cold.
- ☐ Sleep before 10 p.m.
- ☐ Talk about your feelings to someone.

Liver Qi Stagnation

Liver qi stagnation is a stagnation of energy in the liver organ.

Symptoms

Symptoms of liver qi stagnation include:

- a lump in the throat that cannot be swallowed
- anxiety
- better energy levels after exercising
- breast lumps
- cold hands or feet
- cysts
- depression
- feeling low
- feeling wound up
- headaches
- irregular menstrual cycles
- irritability
- menstrual pain
- moodiness
- muscle tension
- pain or distension on the side of the body (the hypochondrium), abdomen or chest
- premenstrual syndrome (PMS)
- regular sighing
- swollen and tender breasts before menstruating
- vertigo

Testing

If you have three or more of the above symptoms, then you may have a stagnation of liver qi.

Causes

In Chinese medicine, the liver is responsible for controlling the menstrual cycle. It is easily affected by frustration or stress, which can lead to anger, resentment and unexpressed emotions. It is the main organ for women and the one that often needs treating to improve fertility.

Trying for a baby is emotionally very stressful, with the highs and lows of the menstrual cycle: low once bleeding starts, then optimistic around ovulation, through to mental anxiety towards the end of the cycle, waiting to see whether you're pregnant. Together with seeing women all around you falling pregnant seemingly easily will create frustration and resentment (liver qi stagnation).

Risks

The risks of having a stagnation of energy in the liver organ include:

- irregular menstrual cycles
- unexplained infertility

Treatment

If you have liver qi stagnation don't worry – most people do. Surrender control, have acupuncture, which is very effective at treating this condition, and, if it's severe, take Chinese herbs and seek out a good fertility counsellor. You can practise a simple breathing exercise to help you. Take a breath in through your nose and say 'I' and breathe out through your mouth and say 'surrender'.

Going out and meeting friends or family will make you feel comforted and is a nice distraction from always thinking about trying for a baby. That doesn't mean you're not taking it seriously enough, or not giving it 100 per cent. Actually, it's the opposite – you need downtime, rest and balance that will greatly benefit your fertility.

Treatment checklist ☑

☐ Exercise three to four times a week.

☐ Have fun and distract yourself from your fertility journey.

☐ Have weekly acupuncture treatment.

☐ Practise yoga, t'ai chi, mindfulness or meditation.

☐ Take Chinese herbs if severe and have counselling.

☐ Watch comedies (laughter therapy).

Blood Stasis

Blood stasis (stagnation) occurs when blood fails to move freely around the body. To use an analogy, blood stasis is like when the water in your house pipes freezes during winter when it gets too cold. The water doesn't move (stasis) and the bursting of the pipes is the point of blood stasis. Sometimes blood stasis can be painful and the bursting of water through the pipes is like the point of pain we feel within our bodies.

Symptoms

Symptoms of blood stasis include:

- absence of a menstrual period (amenorrhoea)
- breast lumps
- clots in the menstrual flow
- dark menstrual blood flow
- endometriosis
- fixed abdominal pain
- headaches
- heavy periods (menorrhagia)
- mental restlessness
- painful periods
- PCOS
- premenstrual pain
- purple nails and lips
- the uterus lining merges with the uterus muscle (adenomyosis)

Testing

If you have three or more of the above symptoms then it's likely you have a stagnation of blood. You may also have a stagnation of qi or a deficiency of qi too. Most people do.

Causes

This is a common condition that can easily be brought on by stress, frustration, excessive exercise, exposure to the cold, poor diet and lifestyle. The causes of blood stasis include:

- a deficiency of blood (anaemia)

- a deficiency of qi (energy)
- excessive cold (yin) inside the body
- stagnation of qi

Risks

If the stasis of blood is left untreated it can slow down the functioning of the body, causing lots of problems, including the formation of lumps in the body. These lumps are hard and painful when touched. Endometriosis and PCOS are all forms of blood stasis. The risks of having blood stasis include:

- ectopic pregnancies
- implantation failure
- myomas (benign tumours)
- painful periods (dysmenorrhoea)
- unexplained infertility

Treatment

The object of treatment is to move the blood. You need more blood, more energy or more heat to move the blood. Improving diet and lifestyle habits can greatly relieve blood stasis and improve your fertility. You can apply a hot water bottle to your lower abdomen before ovulation (not afterwards) to help blood flow to your uterus. Acupuncture is good at moving blood, as it's a great regulator. However, Chinese herbs are often better as they can move blood as well as generate more blood.

Treatment checklist ☑️

☐ Apply heat, such as a hot water bottle, to your lower abdomen, but only if you tend to feel cold and only before you ovulate.

☐ Eat warming foods such as ginger, turmeric and cardamom.

☐ If your feet are cold, use a warm foot spa.

☐ Look at your emotions and see if you need to work through them.

☐ Reduce your energy expenditure: don't exercise more than three times a week, don't work night shifts or work more than 40 hours a week.

☐ Wear enough clothing to keep your body warm as well as warm footwear.

Yin Deficiency

A deficiency of yin is a lack of bodily fluids, for example cervical mucous, seminal fluid or a uterus lining that isn't sticky. Yin is related to youthfulness, fertility and longevity. It is housed in the kidneys.

Symptoms

Night-time is yin while daytime is yang. Sweating at night highlights a deficiency of yin. A woman's body temperature increases from ovulation and rises until either bleeding starts or there is a positive pregnancy test. At this point, some women will feel too hot at night and will sweat. This shows they have too much heat (yang) due to a lack of yin. The sweat itself is attributed to yin, as it's a fluid.

Symptoms of a yin deficiency include:

- absence of a menstrual period (amenorrhoea)
- a lack of cervical mucous
- anxiety
- dry skin or eyes

- early periods
- excessive hair loss
- fatigue
- feeling thirstier in the evening
- feeling warmer in the evening
- heavy periods (menorrhagia)
- lower back pain
- poor sperm motility
- poor sperm viscosity
- premature ejaculation
- prolonged periods
- sweating at night

Testing

If you have three or more of the above symptoms, then you may have a deficiency of yin.

Causes

Leading a hectic life can easily damage yin; going to bed late and getting up early will 'burn the candle at both ends', which is a good analogy of yin being used up and damaged. A poor diet, dieting, overworking, excessive exercising or physical work, semen loss in men and excessive blood loss in women, can all cause a deficiency of yin. It's important to have a lifestyle that maintains yin, not only for fertility, but also for good health, beauty and longevity.

Risks

The risks of having a yin deficiency include:

- a thin uterus lining
- empty follicle syndrome
- implantation failure
- poor follicle growth
- poor sperm quality
- premature ageing
- reoccurring miscarriages
- unexplained infertility

Treatment

People in China today still practise yin-conservation techniques. Building up yin and conserving it is more than just taking supplements and herbs, it's a way of life!

Treatment checklist ☑

- ☐ Cut out alcohol.
- ☐ Cut out all spicy foods.
- ☐ Don't exercise excessively. Instead practise soft exercises, such as yoga or t'ai chi.
- ☐ Don't work more than 40 hours a week.
- ☐ Don't work night shifts.
- ☐ Drink 2 litres (½ gallon) of water a day.
- ☐ Eat lots of seafood (that don't contain mercury, see page 148).
- ☐ Eat regularly and don't diet.
- ☐ For men, don't lose too much semen. Only release it when trying to conceive around ovulation.
- ☐ Go to sleep before 10 p.m.
- ☐ Have weekly acupuncture treatment and take Chinese herbs daily.
- ☐ Take iron supplements (20mg): good amounts of blood helps to restore yin levels.

Yang Deficiency

Yang is like a combination of energy with heat. It helps to maintain movement and keep us warm.

Symptoms

Symptoms of a yang deficiency include:

- early morning loose bowels
- feeling cold and easy to become cold
- impotence
- late periods
- lower back pain
- not wanting to move

- painful periods (dysmenorrhoea)
- pale urine
- poor LH surge
- scanty periods
- tiredness
- unexplained infertility
- wanting to curl up into a ball

Testing

Daytime is yang, especially the morning. Feeling cold at this time highlights a yang deficiency. Otherwise, if you have three or more of the above symptoms, then you may have a deficiency of yang.

Causes

Causes of a yang deficiency include:

- drinking chilled drinks
- eating raw foods like salads or smoothies
- eating uncooked foods
- excessive use of medications
- exposure to the cold
- living in a cold home
- overworking

Risks

If you become too cold, stasis will set in causing irregular levels of hormones circulating in the body. Other risks of a yang deficiency include:

- reoccurring miscarriages
- unexplained infertility

Treatment

People in England used the hot waters in Bath during the seventeenth century as a cure for infertility in women [121]. The reason why it helped with fertility is that bathing the body in hot water helps to improve yang levels and blood flow. Blood is a liquid and is affected by temperature. When it's warmer, it flows better. An increased rate of blood flow improves the regulation of fertility hormones that are contained within the blood and improves the growth of follicles and helps them to mature.

Treatment checklist ☑

☐ Add more spices into your diet.

☐ Don't eat raw or chilled foods.

☐ Don't leave your hair wet after washing it.

☐ Have weekly acupuncture treatment and take Chinese herbs daily.

☐ Reduce your exposure to the cold and drafts including air conditioning units.

☐ Use a hot water bottle on your lower back.

☐ Wear more clothes and thermals.

Jing Deficiency

Jing means 'essence' in Chinese [122]. In men it is their semen and in women their eggs. During pregnancy it nourishes the foetus and after birth controls growth, sexual maturation, fertility and development. It is housed in the kidneys and is inherited from our parents. If they were healthy and strong, then we inherit their strength and fertility, similar to genetics.

Symptoms

The symptoms of a jing deficiency include:

- burnout
- DNA fragmentation
- dry, brittle hair
- chromosome abnormalities
- chronic infertility
- empty follicle syndrome
- failure to enter puberty or delayed puberty
- low anti-Müllerian hormone (AMH) levels

- poor embryo quality
- poor sperm morphology
- translucent teeth
- weak bones

Testing

In Western medicine, jing is closely connected to AMH and semen quality. Testing your AMH levels and semen quality in conjunction with the above symptoms will give you a good idea as to whether you have a deficiency of jing.

Causes

Jing can be damaged by:

- excessive semen loss
- extreme exercising or working
- long periods of working night shifts
- miscarriages or terminations
- overuse of medications
- persistent illegal stimulant drug use
- poor genetics

Risks

The risks of a jing deficiency include:

- birth defects
- chromosome abnormalities
- infertility
- reoccurring miscarriages

Treatment

Jing, yin and blood are all similar and relate to each other. Good amounts of blood will nourish yin and jing. Good amounts of jing are also needed for blood production. It's therefore important to nourish blood, yin and jing for good fertility.

Treatment checklist ☑

- ☐ Don't work more than 40 hours a week.
- ☐ Don't work night shifts.
- ☐ Have afternoon naps.
- ☐ Have weekly acupuncture treatment and take Chinese herbs daily.
- ☐ Practise soft exercises, such as yoga, t'ai chi and qi gong.
- ☐ Rest as much as you can.
- ☐ Sleep before 10 p.m.
- ☐ Take supplements such as royal jelly (100mg), bee pollen (2-5g), coenzyme Q10 (600mg), myo-inositol (250-500mg) and DHEA (25-75mg) (see Chapter Twelve for more on supplements).

Dampness

Dampness is stagnant yin, like a swamp, bog or fog.

Symptoms

Symptoms of dampness include:

- bleeding in between periods
- bloating
- endometriosis
- excessive vaginal discharge
- genital eczema
- greasy skin
- haemorrhoids
- loose or sticky stools
- overweight
- pain and numbness
- painful periods (dysmenorrhoea)
- PCOS
- poor appetite
- poor sperm quality
- water retention

Testing

If you have three or more of the above symptoms, then you may have dampness.

Causes

The major cause of dampness is diet. Eating gluten, junk food or too much dairy can lead to dampness as the digestive system works harder to process these foods, making it weaker. This weakness reduces fluid metabolism, leading to stagnation of yin, causing dampness. Have you ever wondered why a glass of milk at night helps you to sleep? It's because the spleen finds it hard to process milk as it's damp, making it weak. If the spleen becomes weakened, we feel tired, making it easier to sleep.

Damp climates, like that of the UK, Ireland, New Zealand and the west and southeast coasts of America, can make more people suffer from dampness. We often forget that we live in the middle of an ecosystem and are therefore influenced by it. Energy and blood find it harder to move their way through the body in people with internal dampness, like wading through a swamp. This makes energy and blood move slower, causing stagnation.

Dampness can penetrate the body making it feel colder than it really is, hence why it feels colder in areas where it is damp when compared to other areas that are dry and have lower humidity.

Living in a damp room, wearing damp clothes or sitting on damp ground can also lead to dampness. Excessive worrying and antibiotics can weaken the spleen, causing dampness.

If damp is left untreated for a long time it can cause heat. This is because stagnation festers and causes friction, which eventually generates heat. To use an analogy, when there is a traffic jam on the road, you can feel the heat coming off the car engines because the road is stagnated. When there is no traffic and the cars are able to move freely, you don't feel the heat. When damp is mixed with heat, a new syndrome is created called damp-heat, which is a protracted form of damp that is hard to get rid of.

Risks

The risks of dampness include:

- infertility (and unexplained)
- male infertility
- PCOS

Treatment

Changing your diet will have the biggest impact in ridding the body of dampness. This will mean cutting out a lot of normal foods eaten in Western culture, such as gluten (bread, pasta), dairy products, sugar and processed foods. Once these are eliminated from your diet, your body will start to work better, hence why people who cut these foods out of their diet also lose weight.

Treatment checklist ☑

- ☐ Cut out or greatly reduce your dairy intake.
- ☐ Have weekly acupuncture treatment and take Chinese herbs daily.
- ☐ Reduce or cut out gluten and takeaways from your diet.
- ☐ Reduce your exposure to damp environments, both inside buildings and outside.
- ☐ Try to think positively and practise mindfulness or meditation.

Phlegm

Phlegm is a chronic form of dampness. It is stickier than dampness and will obstruct energy and blood flow more. It can take form and produce lumps that are soft, for example in the breasts or over the ovaries [43].

Symptoms

Symptoms of phlegm include:

- a puffy face
- blocked fallopian tubes
- breast lumps
- feeling heavy and sluggish
- fuzzy head
- greasy skin
- obesity
- polyps
- sweaty genitalia
- swollen fingers or toes
- uterus obstructions

Testing

If you have three or more of the above symptoms, then you may have phlegm.

Causes

The main cause of phlegm is a weakened spleen. The spleen is the main organ for transporting and transforming fluids within the body. If it's weakened by worry, poor diet or exposure to damp it will be less able to process the body's fluids and they will accumulate, stagnate and turn into dampness and then into phlegm. Phlegm is heavy and will sink to the bottom of the body, causing blockages and masses around the reproductive organs.

Risks

The risks of developing phlegm include:

- cysts, fibroids and polyps
- ectopic pregnancies
- infertility
- PCOS

Treatment

Unlike damp, changes to your diet will not be enough to rid the body of phlegm. Other things such as regular exercise, acupuncture and Chinese herbs will be needed to strongly move the stagnation and strengthen the spleen.

> **Treatment checklist** ☑
>
> ☐ Avoid worrying by trying to be in the now; meditating or mindfulness will help with this.
>
> ☐ Cut out dairy, bananas, avocados, lamb and gluten.
>
> ☐ Exercise three to four times a week.
>
> ☐ Have weekly acupuncture treatment and take Chinese herbs daily.
>
> ☐ Try to avoid exposing your body to any wet or damp environments.

Excessive Yang (Heat)

An excess of yang is the same as having too much heat inside your body.

Symptoms

Symptoms of excessive yang include:

- anxiety
- dark urine
- headaches
- heavy periods (menorrhagia)
- hot at night
- irritability
- red face
- restless sleep
- reduced sperm motility
- stressed
- sweating at night
- thirst
- vertigo

Testing

If you have three or more of the above symptoms, then you may have an excess of yang.

Causes

Men are more likely to suffer from this condition than women. This is because men are yang in Nature and tend to consume a lot of yang-type foods and drink, such as red meat, chilli and alcohol. Introducing more yang into the body than we need from excessive consumption of alcohol, red meat, coffee, sugar and spicy food (chilli), substances such as smoking (breathing in of fire), will increase the amount of yang in the body, which will in turn burn and damage yin, making the body cook itself from the inside.

A good example of excessive yang is seen in male chefs. The environment they work in is hot and stressful, which both create heat. Their testicles are on the same level as a cooker or a hot plate, which exposes them to too much heat. A hot environment and direct exposure to a cooker or hot plate raises the temperature around the testicles, making them too hot to produce sperm properly. Stress creates heat that affects the liver. The liver acupuncture channel travels into the groin, which can move heat from the liver into the groin area, causing the testicles to become too hot, all of which can affect sperm production.

Risks

Excessive yang can affect both male and female fertility:

- a lack of cervical mucous
- poor sperm motility
- reoccurring miscarriages
- unexplained infertility

Treatment

Dietary changes will have the biggest impact on most people. Cutting out alcohol, sugar, chilli and red meat will greatly reduce excessive yang being poured into the body. Clearing the excessive heat already in the body will take time. Chinese herbs are particularly good at clearing heat from the body quickly. Reducing stress will also reduce heat in the body.

Treatment checklist ☑

☐ Avoid very hot baths or showers, cookers, heated car seats, laptops and hot environments such as kitchens, saunas, sunbeds and sunbathing.

☐ Cut down on black tea (English tea), coffee, alcohol, red meat and sugar.

☐ Cut out chilli and, if chronic, then milder spices too, such as cinnamon, paprika and turmeric.

☐ Have weekly acupuncture treatment and take Chinese herbs daily.

☐ Reduce exposure to stressful situations.

Excessive Yin (Cold)

An excess of yin means too much cold, dampness or phlegm.

Symptoms

Symptoms of excessive yin include:

- abdominal pain
- anxiety
- cold hands and feet, or the whole body
- excessive sweating
- feeling cold
- loose stools
- pain
- pale urine
- PCOS

Testing

If you have three or more of the above symptoms, then you may have excessive yin.

Causes

Too much cold can be caused by a lack of yang, qi, blood or exposure to the cold. Not only did the ancient people of Asia know of the adverse effects of the cold, so did the ancient Greeks. Hippocrates of

Cos recorded its adverse effects on men in 5BCE: 'From the cold and tiredness they forget their sexual drive and their desire to come into union with the other sex'; about women, he stated, '... nor is their menstrual discharge such as it should be, but scanty and at too long intervals' [123]. This is the same in Chinese medicine.

Cold affects blood, as blood is a liquid. Cold causes the thyroid to overwork in order to keep the body warm, which can cause infertility. In addition, your fertility hormones are transported in your blood, and a reduced rate of blood flow will cause a slowing of hormones, leading to a possible hormone imbalance and infertility. Research has shown that exposure to a cold environment can delay follicular development and cause a low response of the ovaries to FSH as well as be a cause of PCOS [124].

Modern air-conditioned offices can make the air too cold, which can affect blood flow and damage yang, causing colds and infertility. People whose heritage is derived from hotter climates are more likely to suffer from excessive cold when living in colder climates.

Cold can enter the body through the pores of the skin, sweat glands, acupuncture channels and orifices, such as the vagina. It is therefore important to wear clothing to protect yourself against the cold invading your body and damaging your fertility. The term 'catching a cold' literally refers to exposing the body to cold that invades (catching) and damages health. Wearing trousers instead of skirts in winter can help to protect the uterus from cold invasion. When the temperature outside is below 10°C (50°F), wearing thermals helps to keep heat in and the cold out.

Eating foods that are cold, such as salads, ice cream, ice, chilled drinks and sandwiches, can introduce cold into the body.

Risks

The risks of a yin excess include:

- poor foetal growth
- prolonged infertility
- reoccurring miscarriages

Treatment

Wearing enough clothing will have the greatest impact on this problem. Unfortunately, female fashion isn't always good for health and fertility! Add spices to your diet and always drink warm fluids.

Treatment checklist ☑

- ☐ Avoid cold foods like salads, smoothies, chilled sandwiches or cold drinks.
- ☐ Avoid exposure to cold environments.
- ☐ Drink warm fluids.
- ☐ Eat warming foods such as ginger, chilli and cinnamon.
- ☐ Have weekly acupuncture treatment and take Chinese herbs daily.
- ☐ If your feet are cold, use a warm foot spa.
- ☐ Use a hot water bottle on your lower back.
- ☐ Use an electric blanket at a low temperature at night before bed.
- ☐ Wear more clothes and possibly thermals.
- ☐ Wear slippers at home and shoes that keep your feet well covered and warm when outside (no trainers, pumps or sneakers).

Part Three

How to Improve Your Fertility

Bringing a child into the world is life-changing. Getting ready to have a child can also mean changes. These changes are whatever is needed to enhance your fertility and get you your baby. Most likely it will be lots of small changes, but it may involve some big ones too. With big changes, it is important to remember priorities in life: what's most important and what to focus upon. I often see couples wanting to have the baby; the successful career; the toned, fit body; the clean and flawless house… In truth, everything their own way. This is the mind wanting everything to be perfect. However, this perfectionism is unrealistic and wears the body out, which damages fertility.

There needs to be some compromise. Priorities need to be listed and, in some instances, sacrifices need to be made in order to get you your baby. In most men and women this can mean changing their diet, working fewer hours, going to bed early, giving up takeaway foods, drinking less alcohol, or exercising more or less, etc. With some women it may even mean working part-time or giving up work completely to replenish the body enough to have a baby. Everyone is different; some will need to make a few changes and others more. To know what changes you need to make, you first need to understand and listen to your body.

Prepping your body, mind and emotions can play an important role in improving your fertility. Essentially, the mind lives in the future; the body lives in the past; and the emotions are in the now. The key to a healthy life and good fertility is to bring these three aspects of yourself into the present moment, which is where we all live. You are then harmonised. You will be fully functional, with a better regulation of your hormones, without losing energy from your past or future. And because of this, your present moment will be more enriched, more joyful and your fertility will be enhanced.

I would recommend prepping your body, and that of your partner, for at least 3–6 months before trying to conceive. This should give you enough time to detox the body, reenergise yourself and reduce any deficiencies or excesses you may have. Taking time to prep, like with most things in life, helps with the end result. By prepping yourself, you greatly increase the chances of falling pregnant naturally and improving the health of your baby. Research conducted in Australia found that improving your lifestyle and diet together with acupuncture and Chinese herbs for four months was twice as effective as IVF treatment [125].

Chapter 7

Prepping Your Body

The body tends to live in the past. Our bodies store life's trauma and stresses, like data on a hard drive, which can stay with us in our muscles and organs and cause health problems. For example, you may have gone through a period of extreme stress in your life, which would have increased the amount of the stress hormone cortisol in your body that in turn interfered with the production of fertility hormones that led to an irregular menstrual cycle, heavy periods, muscle tension and unexplained infertility.

The emotional stresses that you carry around with you in your body need to be resolved and released in order to stop them blocking you from having a baby. Acupuncture and counselling are good at releasing emotional stresses from the body, thereby aiding better hormone regulation and fertility. You can also do this with mindfulness and meditation. If you find it difficult to meditate by yourself you can join a class or download an app onto your smartphone.

Listening to your body is important when trying for a baby. It helps you learn what your body needs to improve your fertility and when it's the right time to try and conceive. Most people are unaware of their own bodies, for example when they ovulate, details of their menstrual cycle and even their energy levels. The mind seldom becomes tired which tricks people into thinking that their energy levels are good. An overactive mind can weaken the body. If we unplug our awareness from our mind and plug it into our body, we can hear what it's saying and what it needs. Exercises such as mindfulness are a great way of getting our awareness to reconnect with our bodies.

The body gives off lots of little signs, which were listed in Chapter Six (page 87), that, when joined together, become a pattern that allows you to see what's going on inside your body. Looking out for these signs makes you become more aware of what your body needs in order to have a baby. It's a learning curve that is also empowering, because awareness of your body helps you to be more aware of who you are. This comes with practice and becomes progressively deeper as we learn and become more self-aware.

When you move into a new house, you first make sure it can protect you from the environment outside, that it's warm, doesn't have damp and has water. It therefore makes sense to prepare your uterus for your baby to call home for the next nine months by making sure your uterus is warm enough, has enough energy and blood, isn't damp and is protected from the harshness of the surrounding environment we call Earth. The uterus is a place for your baby to grow and acts as a transitional home, allowing the baby to acclimatise to our world.

Optimising your lifestyle is an easy way to take control of your fertility and take proactive steps to improve your chances of having your baby. We are often told that a good lifestyle is to lose weight (on the latest celebrity diet) and to exercise (like a marathon runner), while still going to work, having the successful career, dressed in the latest fashions, having a lovely clean house, being a great cook and a social bunny. From a Chinese medicine point of view, trying to achieve all of this depletes energy and blood. This leads to reduced levels of leptin and irregular hormone levels that can cause infertility.

To enhance fertility, energy and blood levels need to be increased.

You should save and bank your energy rather than spend it, in order to get your body out of 'fertility debt'. You can help your uterus become a better home by changing the way you eat, what you eat, the amount of time you sleep, the amount you exercise, the amount of time you spend at work and the type of clothes you wear to ensure good amounts of energy and blood are available for your baby.

Sleep

Sleep can greatly affect fertility. Going to sleep near midnight or afterwards damages yin as midnight is the highest point of yin. This can affect egg and sperm quality. There is a saying: 'Two hours before midnight is worth 10 after.' I couldn't agree more! Those two hours before midnight safeguards your yin for your fertility. To enhance your fertility, try not to go to sleep later than 10 p.m. It will take some practice if you're not used to it, but you'll notice how much better you will feel for it. Research has shown that women who work in the evenings or do night shifts have fewer eggs available [126]. This is because their jing is drained from excessive yin loss.

Research has shown that women who sleep 7–8 hours a night have better fertility [127], while women who sleep 4–6 hours and those that sleep 9–11 hours have reduced fertility. Sleeping for 4–6 hours reduces the amount of energy, blood, leptin and melatonin in the body, thereby damaging fertility, while women who need 9–11 hours of sleep a night have a deficiency, which means their fertility is already damaged and the body is trying to recover by sleeping more.

Having power naps in the afternoon is a great way of boosting your energy levels and fertility. You only need to nap for 20 minutes to revive your body's energy levels.

Not only is the quantity of time you sleep important but also its quality. The quality of sleep can be affected by anxiety, vivid dreams, urinating at night, noise disturbances or having an uncomfortable bed. Having a comfortable mattress and pillow is critical because you spend so much time using it – on average 26 years of your life sleeping! Invest in ones that you find the most comfortable and will allow you to fall into a deep, dreamless sleep. Dreaming at night is not good in Chinese medicine. It means that your mind is still working, when it really needs the time to shut down and rest, otherwise it can disturb sleep, causing reduced energy and blood levels which damage fertility. If you are sensitive to noise, use ear plugs. If you wake at night to pee, try not to drink any fluids an hour or so before bed. Good sleep is golden!

If you find it hard to sleep or you wake during night or at 5 a.m., then your mind is most likely restless and anxious. Try to wind down before going to bed. Don't watch TV, or use your phone, computer or tablet, for at least one hour before you sleep as a lot of stimuli can keep you awake, especially blue light. Instead read a fictional book, listen to music or practise yoga to stretch out the stresses of the day. This will help you to wind down and relax, making sleep easier.

Baths versus showers

More often than not, women tend to prefer having hot baths while men like warm showers. Having a bath after ovulation is a no-no, as the heat around the uterus can cause a fertilised embryo to dislodge from the uterus wall, causing an early miscarriage. However, it's okay to have a bath before ovulation – just not afterwards. Men also need to be careful how much heat they subject themselves too, especially their groin area. A man's testicles are outside their bodies to keep them cooler for optimal sperm production. Excessive heat in the groin area damages sperm production, motility and the DNA within the sperm head. For these reasons, men should avoid baths altogether and should just have warm showers instead. They should also avoid saunas and Jacuzzis for the same reason.

Having wet hair loses heat (yang) from the head. We have hair on our heads to protect us from the sun and to keep heat in. Dry your hair immediately after washing it and never leave your home with wet hair. Having wet hair can reduce the body's temperature, reduce blood flow and cause the body to use up important energy reserves to keep you warm, which could otherwise be used for your fertility. Being cold can also affect the thyroid causing thyroid-related infertility and the distribution of follicle stimulating hormone (FSH) to the ovaries.

Exercise

Regular exercise is good for both male and female fertility. I would recommend around 30 minutes of cardio (non-impact) activity, such as cycling, rowing or cross-training, three times a week. This helps to regulate energy and blood flow, and reduce stress hormones such as cortisone from within the body that can cause infertility. Impact sports such as running, tennis and badminton may cause an embedded embryo to become dislodged from the uterus wall and miscarry. Softer exercises that help the body to relax should be combined with cardio workouts. For example, exercises such as yoga or Pilates plus cardio three times a week.

Too much exercise is harmful to both male and female fertility. Being fit just means you are fit, it doesn't mean you are healthy! This is a misconception in Western culture. Recent research has shown that women who exercise too much have fewer eggs available [107]. Exercise uses up a lot of the body's resources – qi, blood, yin and jing – leaving fewer left over for fertility.

Often people exercise to give themselves more energy. This works by the heart pumping blood around the body, which regulates its flow and allows the body to clean up any issues it might have, but it doesn't actually give you more energy, it just makes it move around the body better, regulating it, making you feel that you have more energy. Only exercises such as qi gong can actually give you more energy. Otherwise, energy comes from good sleep and good food.

Sedentary lifestyle

New research has shown that men who spend more time sitting down watching TV have lower testosterone levels and sperm counts [128]. This is probably due to the excessive heat that builds up around the testes from sitting down, with no air flow to cool them down. This can be a real problem for gamers. I recommend that men should limit their use of the Internet for gaming and sitting down to a few hours at a time.

Women who lead a sedentary lifestyle are more likely to put on weight, especially around their abdomen, which, in Chinese medicine, can cause stagnation and slows down the regulation of blood flow to the uterus and fertility hormones to the ovaries causing infertility and PCOS.

Pace

Today's modern pace of life does nothing to help fertility. The faster we move or do things, the more energy we use up. It's like having a fast car: a car with a bigger engine and more cylinders uses more petrol (energy), while a car with a smaller engine and fewer cylinders uses less energy. By moving at a fast pace we use up energy and blood that could cause levels of leptin to drop, which will affect the regulation of hormones released by the hypothalamus. If we move at a slower pace and have more patience, we use up less energy and are able to conserve more of it for our fertility.

Drug use

Men should not use any illegal drugs such as cocaine, crack, MDMA or THC for at least six months before trying to conceive as they damage sperm DNA. They drain jing (essence) in Chinese medicine [129] [130], which can also damage egg quality in women.

Both men and women should refrain from smoking cigarettes, including vape inhalers, as nicotine damages semen quality and can prevent a woman from ovulating and impede implantation of the embryo into the uterus wall [68] [69].

I would recommend that both men and women limit their alcohol intake each week to no more than two glasses of red wine (125ml/1.4 units per glass).

Clothing

Clothes and their impact upon fertility are seldom looked at in fertility treatment. In today's world we are often insulated from the Earth's environment. We look out through the window of our temperature-controlled homes and try to predict what the temperature will be like outside.

Wearing the right clothes for the right season can greatly improve your fertility. Research has shown that exposure to the cold affects FSH levels to the ovaries [11]. When the outside temperature is below 10°C (50°F), it's better for your health and fertility to wear thermal undergarments to keep the heat in, especially the legs. Most people will wear three or four layers on their upper body but only one layer on their legs! The legs contain our largest muscle groups and if they get cold it can affect blood flow and the hormones contained within it.

It's important to keep your uterus warm and protect it from the cold. You wouldn't leave the doors or windows open in your baby's nursery to let the cold in, so why would you do it with your uterus? Wearing thermal undergarments when it's cold is like insulating your house from losing heat (energy), keeping your uterus nice and warm and making it a perfect home for your new baby. You can apply a hot water bottle on your lower abdomen before ovulation to help with blood flow to the follicles and uterus. Once you've ovulated, don't apply any heat to your lower abdomen; instead apply it to your lower back if you're cold, which will help your yang and will keep you warm.

There is a saying in old English that goes 'Ne'er cast a clout till May be out', which means don't cast off your winter clothes until the end of May. People fall ill in winter because the coldness slows down blood flow, making the immune system less effective in combating viruses, much like an ambulance stuck in traffic. With the advent of 'modern medicine' over the last century, people have become accustomed to wearing less clothing for the sake of fashion and then using acetaminophen (paracetamol - tylenol) or antibiotics when they fall ill. This isn't good for our health or fertility. Not wearing enough clothes leaks energy that could otherwise be used to increase levels of leptin allowing proper hormone regulation and better fertility.

If you feel too warm, then this too can make your uterus an inhospitable environment for your baby to call home for nine months, which can cause a miscarriage or preterm labour. If you feel too warm, you need to make changes to your diet to cool yourself down and not expose your body to excessive heat, including exercising, stress, saunas and sunbeds.

Men tend to be warmer than women and their testicles can be affected by too much heat. They should wear loose-fitting underwear and trousers that allow air to circulate within them.

Footwear

Shoes and fertility may not be an obvious connection, but wearing the correct footwear can have a big impact upon your health and fertility. Regulating the temperature of your feet is an easy way to regulate your body temperature. Warm feet equals warm body; cold feet equals cold body! Yet, in winter time, people don't always wear covered footwear to keep their feet warm. As I've just said, blood is a liquid; it's affected by temperature. If you have cold feet, it makes the body feel cold and slows down blood flow around the body, including to the uterus, thereby damaging hormone regulation and fertility.

I often criticise my patients for coming into my clinic wearing trainers, sneakers, pumps or boat shoes on their feet in wintertime.

This is because the sole of the shoe isn't thick enough to keep the coldness of the ground away from the foot, so the foot becomes cold. Instead, it's better to wear boots in wintertime to keep the feet protected from the cold ground. Trainers (sneakers) are often made of mesh, which allows air to enter the shoe and cool the foot down when exercising. In wintertime, they let cold air in, which makes the foot cold and damages blood circulation. Only wear trainers when exercising indoors during wintertime or outside in summer time.

It's also important to keep your feet warm while indoors, especially in the winter or in cold buildings or on cold floors. Wearing socks and slippers around the home will help to regulate blood flow around the body and improve hormone regulation and your fertility. If you suffer from very cold feet, I would recommend using a warm foot spa daily to help encourage blood flow and improve your circulation.

Donating blood

Donating blood plays an important role in today's society, which helps other less fortunate people and should be applauded. Without it, many people would die. However, when trying for a baby, conserving and building blood is vitally important in the treatment of infertility. Women lose blood every month and need to rebuild it. But due to stressful lives, careers, excessive exercising, social activities and poor diets, blood levels are often lower than they should be. When trying for a baby, a woman cannot afford to give away any of her blood as it's needed for her fertility, growing the placenta and her baby. Blood donors are more likely to develop an iron deficiency, which can affect fertility and a pregnancy [119]. For these reasons, I do not recommend women donate blood when trying for a baby. However, in the majority of cases, it is okay for men to donate blood while trying for a child as they don't lose blood every month.

Dieting

Often when women come to see me for the first time, they'll say they want to lose weight and have a baby. Sometimes it is necessary to lose some weight if the waist–hip ratio is higher than 0.8 as this improves fertility. In such cases it's best done through exercise and a good diet. Dieting is not advisable as this weakens the body and reduces levels of LH and leptin, which can damage fertility. Instead, follow this simple advice on how to lose weight:

- Acupuncture has been shown in research to help with weight loss [131].

- Cut out gluten – this will help you to lose weight quickly as gluten can impair the spleen's function, weakening it, which causes weight gain.

- Cut out refined sugar from your diet.

- Don't eat too late, i.e. after 7 p.m.

- Eat a good, balanced diet (as shown in Chapter Eleven).

- Eat foods rich in copper as it is important in fat metabolism [132]. Foods high in copper include whole grains, beans, nuts, potatoes, dark leafy greens and dried prunes.

- Exercise (cardio) three times a week, but no more.

If a woman has been dieting and then falls pregnant, the pregnancy is at risk as the body is in a weakened state. In such cases, acupuncture and Chinese herbs are vitally important in supporting the woman and baby, especially in the first 12 weeks.

Improving your menstrual cycle

Improving your menstrual cycle is the most important aspect of infertility treatment for a woman. This lies at the cornerstone of Chinese medicine and is something overlooked by Western medicine. By improving your menstrual cycle, it helps growth and maturation of the egg and its implantation into the wall of the uterus. It also reduces the risk of an early miscarriage by ensuring adequate blood flow to the uterus and hormone regulation.

Here are several steps you can take to improve your menstrual cycle:

1. Rest and don't exercise when you have your period, as it can cause a blood deficiency.

2. Reduce the amount of cosmetics you use to just two or three. For example, just use deodorant and hand/face cream and cut out lipstick, nail polish and perfume. If you are unsure what is in your cosmetics and whether they are safe to use, you can download an app onto your smartphone that will tell you. Search in the app store for 'Think Dirty' or 'Healthy Living'.

3. Getting to sleep early will help your energy levels if they are low during your menstrual bleed. Sleeping before 10 p.m. is ideal and for 7–8 hours.

4. If you crave sweet foods when you've got your period, it's because your body needs quick energy as you're losing energy in the form of blood. This may indicate that you have a blood deficiency. Increase your intake of iron and protein, and make sure you rest.

5. Look at your menstrual blood flow. Is it dark or bright red? Does it have any clots? If it's dark with clots, this is stagnation of blood as it's not moving freely. This may be caused by frustration at not being pregnant or exposure to the cold. Practise mindfulness and use a hot water bottle on your abdomen when bleeding. Get to know your body again!

6. If you have pain, use a hot water bottle or acupuncture rather than painkillers to ease the discomfort. Pain in Chinese medicine is caused by stagnation. Heat helps blood to move, as it's a liquid, thereby helping with the stagnation. This is how acupuncture helps to relieve pain. Painkillers have side effects that can damage fertility.

7. Use moon cups or sanitary towels rather than tampons – sorry! Using a tampon is more likely to cause blood to back up rather

than flow out freely. This can lead to a residue of blood, which forms blood stasis in the uterus. Blood stasis in the uterus can cause problems with growth of the new uterus lining; as well as obstruct sperm getting to the egg. Blood residue can also lead to endometriosis, polyps and fibroids.

8. Keep your abdomen covered so it's not exposed to the cold and is kept warm. This will help the blood move out freely and make your uterus lovely and warm for your new baby to call home.

9. If you find that you are more sensitive to crowds of people or pain during your period, it can highlight a lack of energy. We need to have a certain amount of energy to deal with people and tolerate pain. Take ginseng and iron supplements, and optimise your diet (see Chapters Eleven and Twelve for more on this).

10. If you suffer from premenstrual symptoms such as cramps, pain, PMS and tender breasts, it highlights you are frustrated. Find a quiet space and try to relax, meditate or do mindfulness meditation, or seek out an acupuncturist.

11. Be aware that crossing time zones, for example GMT to PST, may affect the length of your menstrual cycle and when you ovulate.

12. Have acupuncture treatment at least once a week. You may also need to take Chinese herbs.

Improving egg quality

There are three stages in the development of an egg that takes place over 85 days. The three successive stages of egg development are:

1. Mulitplication phase.
2. Growth phase.
3. Maturation phase [40].

During each of these stages, the development and thus the quality of the egg can be affected by the following factors:

- Levels of leptin, which regulate the hypothalamus, pituitary gland and fertility hormones such as FSH and LH. Leptin relates to energy levels. Conserving your energy will increase levels of leptin, improve hormone regulation and egg quality.

- Complex carbohydrates which are needed for the hormone FSH to active follicle growth and assist in its maturation, ovulation and subsequent fertilisation [133] [134]. It's therefore important for egg quality to make sure that the woman eats plenty of complex carbohydrates, around 250–350g per day, see page 165.

- Man-made chemical exposure from cosmetics, smoke, packaging, plastics and food affect hormones in the body and egg quality (see Chapter Four for more on this).

- Road traffic air pollution. Wear an air pollution mask or avoid main roads with heavy traffic or underground trains.

- Lacking enough nutrients, vitamins and minerals. Take a good-quality prenatal supplement (see Chapter Twelve).

- Stress, excessive exercising, working night shifts or lifting heavy objects. Reduce stress, don't work night shifts and practise mindfulness, meditation or yoga.

- Taking acetaminophen (paracetamol - tylenol) or aspirin, which can affect ovulation. Don't take painkillers. Use heat pads, gels, balms or acupuncture instead [135].

You can enhance your egg quality by:

- Avoiding foods that contain soya and caffeine.

- Avoiding substances that contain cadmium and mercury (see page 147-8 for more on this).

- Drinking filtered tap water. Don't reuse plastic bottles.

- Eating good amounts of protein, complex carbohydrates and essential fatty acids (see Chapter Ten for more on this).
- Following my male and female diet plans (see Chapter Eleven).
- Having weekly acupuncture treatment.
- Making sure you have adequate levels of calcium in your diet, which aids the maturation of the egg. Good sources of calcium include: almonds, Brazil nuts, hazelnuts, kelp, nori seaweed, parsley, quinoa, sardines and sunflower seeds.
- Making sure you sleep for 7–8 hours a night.
- Reducing cosmetic use to just two items, i.e. deodorant and hand/face cream.
- Taking a powerful antioxidant, such as melatonin (3mg), before sleeping to protect egg quality.
- Taking Chinese herbs daily (see Chapter Fourteen).
- Taking supplements such as DHEA (25–75mg), coenzyme q10 (600mg) and royal jelly (1000mg) daily.

Improving sperm quality

Improving sperm quality can be largely achieved by changing a man's diet. Cutting out meat, chilli, alcohol (which most men consume in abundance) and cow's milk, and replacing them with fish, algae (spirulina and chlorella) and water has been shown to improve semen quality. Both acupuncture and Chinese herbs can also improve sperm quality.

Men should avoid heat around their groin area, so no laptops on the lap, tight-fitting underwear, saunas or sunbeds. Men should also avoid stress and working long hours and staying up late (past 10 p.m.). Men should eat plenty of foods with antioxidants as they can protect sperm from free radical damage and avoid substances that contain cadmium, lead and mercury (see page 147-8). Supplements that can improve semen quality and should be taken daily include:

- coenzyme q10 (600mg)
- essential fatty acids: omega-3 (14g)
- l-arginine (15g)
- lycopene (5-10mg)
- selenium (200mcg)
- vitamin C (1g) [136]
- vitamin E (100-400mg)
- zinc (15-66mg) [137]

Men should avoid excessive semen loss as this can weaken the body. Ideally, semen should only be ejaculated when trying for a baby around ovulation.

Improving implantation

Implantation is controlled by several factors: the embryo, the mother's immune system, levels of leukaemia inhibitory factor (LIF) and advanced glycation end products (AGEs). LIF is a cytokine (immune messenger) that helps regulate immune function in the uterus, while AGEs are proteins or lipids that bond to sugars, which can make the uterus lining inhospitable to an embryo.

- Ensuring a good-quality embryo (see above) will help the embryo hatch and start its implantation into the mother's uterus wall.

- Implantation only takes place during the limited 'implantation window', a 4–5 day period when the uterus is receptive, between days 20 and 24 of a regular menstrual cycle [62]. The mother's immune system retreats (levels of TH1 drop) after ovulation allowing an embryo to implant [62]. However, if the woman has higher than normal levels of the immune cell TH1 in her body, the embryo won't be able to implant. Acupuncture can regulate levels of TH1/TH2 and increase levels of LIF, which are both needed for normal implantation [62] [64].

- Being relaxed and not stressed can also reduce immune factors that can affect the embryo implanting.

- Eating plenty of essential fatty acids, such as omega-3, helps to regulate immune function, thereby allowing the embryo to implant into the uterus wall [138].

- Consuming fewer foods and fluids with sugar can reduce levels of AGEs which affects implantation [1].

- Taking ginseng supplements can increase levels of TH2, which protects an embryo implanting into the uterus lining [336].

Chapter 8

Prepping Your Mind and Emotions

We've talked a lot about the body and fertility, but the mind and emotions can play an equally important role in fertility. The mind has evolved to keep us alive – it's our greatest survival tool. It helps us plan and problem-solve, which helped us survive thousands of years ago in the wild. It doesn't like surprises; they make it agitated, which manifests as anxiety. It likes life to be predictable, which makes it feel secure and for this reason it likes control. In today's world, our minds are overused. We all worry about what's to come and try to plan for our future, education, career, pensions, etc. For most people, their mind is focused on controlling the future.

Our emotions live in the now. They react to what we believe about our life, what we've been told is the truth. Our emotions are constantly bubbling at the surface, mixing with thoughts and stored traumas held within the body from our past. Emotions lie at the heart of trying for a baby. Wanting a baby reveals a very deep-rooted emotional need. Emotions can be high and low during the menstrual cycle when trying naturally. For example, a lot of women feel emotionally low when their menstrual cycle starts, because they are not pregnant. They then pick themselves up and think positively towards ovulation and say to themselves 'It will be this cycle!' Once ovulation has occurred, feelings of anxiety and doubt creep in with questions such as 'Am I, aren't I pregnant?', leading up to the end of the menstrual cycle.

Having fertility challenges can cause a lot of anxiety. Anxiety, like stress, is a negative emotion that serves little positive purpose and simply drains the body of important energy and blood reserves, making it weaker, which damages fertility. The more anxious we are, the more we 'spend' energy and the worse our fertility becomes. It's therefore important to control your mind.

In Chinese medicine, each internal organ is associated with a particular emotion: emotional upset, frustration and anger will affect the liver organ; worrying will damage the spleen; fear weakens the kidneys; and anxiety the heart.

It is difficult not to get emotional when trying for a baby. Often people will say, 'Just relax and let it happen.' If only relaxing was that easy! Most people find it hard to relax in today's modern world. Instead of trying to force yourself to relax and tame your emotions, which is very difficult, I recommend that you have fun instead. Watching comedies, going out for lunch or dinner, to the cinema, shopping with friends, etc., all help to distract you from feeling stressed and anxious and bring joy back into your life and joy is the opposite of anxiety. Happiness helps the body to relax and that in turn helps the flow of energy and blood in the body. This helps regulate the hormones and menstrual cycle, and improves fertility. Research has shown that acupuncture treatment can reduce infertility-related stress [139].

Research has finally proven what Eastern philosophies have known for centuries – that these stresses and emotions can be passed on to our children through our genes [140]. This in turn acts as an emotional disability, which the child inherits and is burdened to resolve in order to have a happy life. Resolving negative emotions before conceiving your baby gives your child a head start, an easier life, with fewer emotional issues for them to work through.

When trying to conceive, most people will start to take supplements to nourish their body and improve their fertility, overlooking their mind and emotions. If the mind and emotions are left unchecked, they consume energy and blood, making the body weaker, which can reduce levels of leptin and damage hormone regulation, even though you may be taking supplements for energy and blood. In order to improve fertility, it's important to prep your mind and emotions as well as your body. It's often harder to prep the mind and emotions, as we tend to be unaware of them. Talking about how we feel or what our fears are, forms part of the way we can prep the mind and emotions and improve our fertility. This can be with friends, family, online forums (**www.myfertilityforum.com**), your doctor, your acupuncturist or a trained professional, such as a fertility counsellor. Once the negative emotion is talked about, aired, given space and confronted, it will dissolve and will not continue to drain your body of vital energy and blood that could otherwise be used for your fertility.

You are not your mind; you are your awareness that sits behind the mind. By taking a step back mentally and watching what you're thinking, you can identify thoughts that could be blocking you from having a baby. For example, negative thought patterns, worrying and anxiety are all diseases of the mind. These diseases then initiate hormonal changes in the physical self which can cause infertility.

Taking a step back from your thoughts and watching them takes time and practice. Just as you need to exercise your muscles at the gym, you need to do the same with your mind, but instead of making your mind bigger, like making a muscle bigger at the gym, you need to do the opposite and make it smaller. This can be achieved through various techniques, such as meditation, mindfulness, yoga, t'ai chi or simply walking in Nature. You can then identify any negative thought patterns you might have and look to see where they originate from and change them. For example, a negative thought pattern about your infertility may be rooted in a belief that you are not 'good enough' to be a parent or feel emotionally or financially unready.

Your mind is like a garden: what you plant (think) is what you grow (feel). Removing negative thoughts and beliefs is like removing weeds from your garden. Learning more about yourself and changing negative thought patterns to become a better person, and therefore a better parent, is one of the silver linings of struggling with infertility.

Reducing stress, building up your strength and having fun!

Stress is one of the greatest causes of infertility [19] [141] [142] [143] [144] [145]. It creates frustration, resentment and even anger, which increase levels of cortisol in the body that affects the normal balance of fertility hormones. This in turn affects the liver organ causing an irregular menstrual cycle, thereby damaging fertility.

Prolonged stress (more than a few hours) weakens the body. As we've seen, the body has three levels of stress:

1. The alarm phase (level 1).
2. The resistance phase (level 2).
3. The exhaustion phase (level 3) [30].

Most people live in the resistance phase (level 2). The resistance phase causes an increase in adrenal hormone release (glucocorticoids), which causes an increase in energy demands and reduces reserves of lipids and levels of leptin. Lipids are made up of fats and oils and are yin in nature. These form the foundations of good health and fertility. It's therefore important to have a diet rich in essential fatty acids, such as those from oily fish or flaxseed, to maintain high levels of lipids and offset the side effects of stress. Often people are recommended to eat high levels of protein for fertility, but this isn't enough. High levels of omega-3s are equally as important. They also help to regulate the immune system and implantation.

Prolonged stress can affect your immune system, causing an increase in cortisol levels, which reduce the number of TH2 cells. TH2 cells are important in supporting an implanting embryo into the uterus [145]. Chronic stress can cause the prolonged release of cortisol, against which white blood cells mount a counter-regulatory response by down-regulating their cortisol receptors. This down-regulation reduces the cells' capacity to respond to anti-inflammatory signals and allows cytokine-mediated inflammatory processes to flourish, increasing levels of TH1 cells. Having greater numbers of TH1 cells can prevent the embryo from implanting into the uterus wall.

Acupuncture is very good at reducing stress by regulating levels of the stress hormone cortisol and by regulating the hypothalamus, both of which regulate fertility hormones and the menstrual cycle [146]. The combination of having acupuncture and lying on the treatment couch encourages people to relax. Together with heat and relaxing music, the person is sent into a deep state of relaxation. In this state, the body is no longer in the resistance phase and is able to let go, and has a chance to heal itself back to a state of balance.

When trying for a baby, most women will be proactive; they will do their research and try everything to have a baby. However, trying too hard can cause stress and anxiety, which increases levels of stress hormones, which cause an irregular menstrual cycle and also use up important energy that could have been used for fertility. I sometimes have to tell my patients not to try so hard, and relax. Having fun will help reduce stress, improve blood flow, improve your menstrual cycle and aid fertility. Trying all the techniques in this book is important, and will greatly increase your chances of having a baby, but do so up to a point where it doesn't cause you stress. Beyond that it can become a hindrance. When that happens, remember to surrender, let your hair down and have fun. Energy and blood flows better when you're happy.

And if blood flows better, your hormones will flow better and your fertility will be better.

Vision boards

You can use a 'vision board' to help your fertility. A vision board is where you put positive images onto a board for you to look at each day, for example a positive pregnancy test, a baby, you and your partner holding a baby, a cot, a buggy, etc. Looking at these images each day allows you to bring them into your life, to accept them as part of your reality and that they are true to you.

Vision boards are also a useful way of seeing inside yourself and finding any emotional blocks that you might have about having a baby. For example, if you look at your vision board and don't believe it, then trace this negative thought back to where it originates from and confront it to change it. You can do this by sitting in a quiet room and analysing your thoughts – watch them and see where they lead to.

What we think is determined by how we feel about ourselves and what we believe. If we think we aren't good enough or a failure, then the body will listen to this and make it so. In Chinese medical terms, believing you're a failure or not good enough lowers your energy levels, causing a reduction in the creation of energy and blood, stagnates the liver qi causing blood stasis, which leads to an irregular menstruation that's painful and damages the kidney qi, which affects egg and sperm quality. Believe in yourself!

Being positive

Generally, negative thought patterns come from a negative belief we have about ourselves, for example 'I'm not good enough' or 'I don't deserve it.' These beliefs are rooted in fear and not in the love of yourself. To change this you can use positive affirmations such as 'I love myself' or 'I am pregnant' or 'I surrender' if you're stressed. Take five minutes now to practise one of these techniques. Take a breath in and say 'I' and a breath out and say one of the affirmations above, for example 'am pregnant'. Breath is a useful affirmation tool as the in breath is a state of wanting to be alive here on this planet while the out breath forms the surrender to the belief of what you are saying.

Research has shown that women who are negative about their fertility are more likely to fail [147]. Reducing your exposure to negative influences is important, and that means not spending time with negative people, or watching horror movies or negative documentaries, and not watching or reading negative news. Instead watch comedies, positive news or read light-hearted novels that allow your mind to switch off from always thinking about negative things and puts you in a positive state of mind.

Chapter 9

Optimising Your Environment

We are becoming more aware of our impact upon the environment but seldom think how this affects our ability to conceive. Everything is connected to each other. For example, the plastics that pollute our oceans also affect our hormones, causing infertility. Understanding how our environment affects our fertility will help you to understand how it affects Nature. We are a part of Nature. If we damage Nature, we damage ourselves.

Reducing your exposure to chemicals

Our bodies are surrounded by around 80,000 chemicals, from fragrances in soaps, shampoos and perfumes to make-up and cleaning products as well as sanitary products such as tampons [148]. Unknowingly this affects our health and fertility. It's better for your fertility and that of your future baby to limit the amount of chemicals in your home (including your garden) and in your body. For example, it's best to have natural flooring in your home rather than carpets, which contain stain-repellent chemicals.

Below are chemicals that are known to affect male and female fertility. These lists aren't conclusive, as most of the 80,000 chemicals in our environment have yet to be tested on human reproductive health.

Chemicals that affect female fertility

These chemicals have been shown in research to damage female fertility:

- 8-prenylnaringenin
- aniline
- anthraquinones
- BPA
- BPS
- DDE
- DDT
- deoxymiroestrol
- dibenzofurans
- hexachlorobenzene
- miroestrol
- octamethylcyclotetrasiloxane
- organophosphate
- PAHs
- parabens
- particulate matter (PM$_{2.5}$)
- PCBs
- PFCs
- PFOA
- PFOS
- phthalates
- polychlorinated biphenyls
- polychlorinated dibenzodiozins

Chemicals that affect male fertility

These chemicals have been shown in research to damage male fertility:

- aniline
- APEs
- DDD
- DDE
- DDT
- parabens
- PBDE
- PCBs
- PFCs
- PFOA
- PFOS
- phthalates
- THC

Know your plastics

The use of plastics is a growing problem, not only for the environment but also for male and female fertility. Plastics are categorised according to their content and recyclability. The recycling symbol number is the code that shows what type of plastic was used to make the product. Plastics with recycling symbols 2, 4 and 5 are generally considered okay to use (see below). Avoid plastics with recycling symbols 3 and 6. Plastics with recycling symbol 7 are okay to use as long as they also say 'PLA' or have a leaf symbol on them. Recycling symbol 1 is okay to use, but shouldn't be used more than once (don't refill plastic water bottles for example). Keep all plastic containers out of the heat and sun as these can cause the chemicals within them to be released into your food and fluids. Always try to buy foods that are not prepacked in plastic and use paper bags to pack loose fruit and vegetables.

Plastic codes

1. Polyethylene terephthalate (PETE or PET): includes clear plastic water and soft drink bottles. Generally considered okay to use, but don't reuse them.

2. High-density polyethylene (HDPE): includes opaque milk jugs, detergent bottles, juice bottles, butter tubs and toiletry bottles. Generally considered okay to use.

3. Polyvinyl chloride (PVC): includes cling film (food wrap), cooking oil bottles and plumbing pipes. Do not cook food in these plastics and try to minimise using them around any type of food (use wax paper, parchment paper or glass containers instead of cling film). Avoid where possible!

4. Low-density polyethylene (LDPE): includes grocery bags, some cling films, squeezable bottles and bread bags. Generally considered okay to use.

5. Polypropylene (PP): includes most yoghurt pots, tea bags, water bottles with a cloudy finish, medicine bottles, and sauce and syrup bottles. Generally considered okay to use.

6. Polystyrene/Styrofoam: includes disposable foam plates, cups and packing materials. Do not cook food or put hot food onto these plastics. Avoid where possible!

7. All other plastics not included in the other categories and with mixes of plastics 1 to 6 are labelled with a 7. Polylactic acid (PLA) is a plastic made from plants that is also labelled with a 7. PLA plastics don't contain BPA, which are bad (see below). No safety concerns have been raised about using PLA plastic with food. It's difficult to tell the difference between a PLA number 7 plastic and a BPA-containing number 7 plastic. Do not cook food in plastics that aren't PLA and avoid using these plastics around any type of food. Office water coolers tend to use reusable plastic bottles made from polycarbonate, number 7, which contain BPAs. Avoid where possible!

BPAs

Bisphenol A (BPA) was first synthesised in 1891, as a synthetic oestrogen. It is now used to make plastic hard, coat paper (till receipts) and to line tins and lids of foods and drinks [85]. BPA can disrupt male and female hormones and has been linked to autism. Products that may contain BPAs include:

- plastic cups, plastic cooking utensils and plastic dishes
- knives, forks and chopsticks
- water bottles, cups and food storage containers
- food processors and blenders (plastic containers and lids)
- tinned foods (BPA is in the liners in nearly every tin)
- takeaway hot beverage cups, i.e. coffee (BPA is in the lining)

Here's how to avoid exposing yourself to BPAs:

- Avoid any plastics with recycling numbers 3, 6 or 7.
- Avoid plastic water bottles. Use filtered tap water and refill metal or glass reusable water bottles.
- Cover food with parchment paper rather than cling film (plastic wrap) or kitchen foil [331].
- Do not drink a hot beverage from a takeaway cup.
- Do not microwave or heat anything in plastic.
- Do not pour any hot liquids into plastic.
- Do not put hot food into plastic containers.
- Reduce your use of tinned foods.
- Use glass, porcelain or stainless steel containers to hold and store food.

Air conditioning

Most office or retail buildings are air-conditioned. People often overlook air conditioning units and their impact upon health and fertility. If you know someone who sits in an office underneath an air conditioning outlet, chances are they've been ill a dozen times. The old saying of 'Stay out of draughts or you'll catch a chill' is still very true today. And a cold is something we get when we're cold. The cold weakens the body, as it needs to use up energy (qi) to keep us warm. The coldness causes blood flow to slow down. A reduced blood flow affects the regulation of fertility hormones which are moved around in the blood. Using more energy to keep warm reduces the amount of energy and blood available for fertility, reduces leptin levels and can make the uterus too cold. A cold uterus can lead to unexplained infertility, endometriosis, adenomyosis (where the lining of the uterus breaks through the muscle wall of the uterus) and reoccurring miscarriages.

The same is true if the air conditioning is set at a high temperature. It can cause irregular thyroid function, excessive sweating, which loses yin, agitation and irritability, which can affect the menstrual cycle.

Reducing your exposure to air pollution

According to the World Health Organization (WHO), over 90 per cent of the world's population lives in areas where air pollution exceeds safety guidelines [149]. More and more research is showing the harmful effects of air pollution upon our health. It's well known that air pollution affects the respiratory system causing people to develop problems with their breathing, such as asthma, but it's less well known how air pollution affects fertility.

Research is now showing how exposure to fine particles known as $PM_{2.5}$ affects both male and female fertility [150] [151] [152]. These particles come from heavy industry, the burning of fossil fuels and car exhaust emissions, especially diesel.

Men who are exposed to air pollution are at a greater risk of developing oxidative stress (see page 72). Sperm are very susceptible to oxidative stress, causing damage to the DNA housed in the sperm head. This can cause chromosome abnormalities in the foetus and an increase in miscarriages and birth defects.

Women who are exposed to air pollution have altered functioning TH2 cells, which may have an impact upon implantation and fertility (see page 52). Exposure to road traffic pollution can reduce female fertility, pregnancy rates and antral follicle counts (AFC) [153].

It's therefore best to avoid exposing yourself to air pollution while trying for a baby or when pregnant. Avoid walking next to busy roads, standing at junctions, using the underground (metro) system or breathing in any type of combustion (cigarette, BBQs, fires) smoke. If you can't avoid being exposed to air pollution, you can protect yourself in three ways:

1. Early research has shown that high doses of B vitamins – B_9 (2.5mg), B_6 (50mg) and B_{12} (1mg) – can reduce the harmful effects of air pollution upon the body [151].

2. Wear an air pollution mask. There are plenty on the market, which offer styles and tastes for all with military grade filtration.

3. Change your car for one that is more environmentally friendly, i.e. one without a diesel engine and that has some form of electric propulsion.

Reducing your exposure to heavy metals

Exposure to heavy metals can damage both male and female fertility and cause birth defects. Heavy metals can increase the number of free radicals in the body, which damage sperm and eggs, and affect implantation. It has long been suggested that at least half the cases of human male infertility of unknown aetiology may be attributable to exposure from various heavy metals [154]. The most important heavy metals that can affect fertility are listed below.

Cadmium (Cd)

The heavy metal cadmium is a pollutant commonly seen in modern industrial processes, for example the burning of fossil fuels and the manufacture of nickel–cadmium batteries. Cadmium is absorbed in significant quantities from cigarette smoke and shellfish, i.e. oysters [156]. A single cigarette contains 2.8 µg of cadmium [155].

Cadmium is known to have numerous undesirable effects upon health in people, targeting the kidneys, liver and arteries and veins in particular, as well as inducing oxidative stress (free radicals). Concentrations of cadmium in the ovaries increase with age and have been associated with failure of egg development from primary to secondary stage, failure to ovulate, implantation failure, early pregnancy loss and birth defects [156].

Leydig cells, which are found in the male testes and produce testosterone that's needed for sperm production, are very sensitive to cadmium [154]. Cadmium has a strong toxic effect upon sperm and can affect sperm density, motility, viability and morphology[154]. Nutritional deficiency in essential elements, such as zinc, may further aggravate the effects of cadmium [154].

Lead (Pb)

Lead can be found in all parts of our environment – the air, soil, water and even inside our homes in a wide variety of different products, including paint, ceramics, pipes and plumbing materials, toys, batteries, ammunition and even cosmetics. Much of our exposure comes from human activities including the burning of fossil fuels and past use of leaded petrol and some types of industrial facilities.

Lead is a well-known toxic metal that can damage human health. Studies have shown it can damage male semen, leading to reduced fertility, birth defects and delayed conception [157]. In women, exposure to lead can increase the risk of miscarrying [158]. Lead can accumulate in our bodies over time, where it is stored in bones along with calcium. During pregnancy, the baby takes half the mother's calcium and is exposed to stored lead [158].

Mercury (Hg)

Low doses of mercury have been shown to decrease male and female fertility [159]. Mercury is found in fish high up in the food chain, such as tuna, swordfish, king mackerel, lobster, Spanish mackerel, marlin, grouper and shark. Research has shown that a diet high in these fish showed a reduced fertility rate in males [160]. High levels of mercury are also found in the air from coal smoke and acid rain. High levels of mercury reduce the absorption of zinc, which can affect sperm production. Cattle kept in an area that has ground water contaminated with mercury can pass this onto humans in their meat [161]. In women, mercury has been shown to affect levels of lymphocytes and natural killer cells, causing immune-type infertility [161].

Reducing your exposure to electromagnetic waves (EMWs)

In today's modern world we are constantly being bombarded with EMWs, from radio, phone masts, wireless devices, etc. Research has shown a correlation between increased mobile (cellular) phone use and reduced male fertility [162] [163]. Semen analysis of mobile phone users showed a decrease in sperm count, motility, viability and normal morphology. The more mobile phone use there was, the greater the damage to semen. This may be caused by several mechanisms:

1. An EMW-specific effect.

2. A thermal molecular effect (too much heat from the phone around the groin area).

3. Susceptibility of Leydig cells, which produce testosterone, to EMW.

4. EMW-dependent decrease in melatonin – an antioxidant – can predispose sperm to reactive oxidative stress (free radicals).

In women, mobile phones can affect thyroid function, causing irregular levels of TSH, which may lead to infertility [164].

Studies have shown that men who use a laptop connected to the Internet via Wi-Fi to surf the net for more than four hours a day can have a significant decrease in sperm progressive motility with an increase in non-motile sperm and a significant increase in sperm DNA fragmentation [165], which can lead to infertility and reoccurring miscarriages. This can be a problem for men who work at a desk job and spend their free time gaming. Levels of EMW are likely to increase with the introduction of 5G.

You can protect yourself from EMWs by either reducing your use of gadgets that emit EMWs or by buying items that neutralise them, i.e. semi-precious stones such as tourmaline [166]. I would recommend turning off your Wi-Fi box (router) at night.

Reducing your exposure to medications

Most people are unaware that commonly used medications can affect fertility. It's important to know which ones can inhibit fertility and the alternatives to use instead.

Painkillers

Painkillers such as acetaminophen (paracetamol - tylenol), acetylsalicylic acid (aspirin) and nonsteroidal anti-inflammatory drugs (NSAIDs, such as ibuprofen and indomethacin) can interfere with male and female fertility. In men, paracetamol, aspirin and indomethacin reduce the amount of testosterone produced, which then affects the production of sperm [167]. Paracetamol use has been shown in research to affect male fertility by delaying time to pregnancy [88].

In women, nonsteroidal anti-inflammatory drugs (NSAIDs) and aspirin have adverse effects on hormone regulation (GnRH), ovulation and fertilisation [168] [169]. For example, diclofenac was the highest inhibitor of ovulation compared to naproxen and etoricoxib. Paracetamol can prevent a woman from ovulating [91]. Drugs such as aspirin and NSAIDs can reduce the pineal gland's production of melatonin by 75 per cent [170], which can affect egg and sperm quality.

For these reasons, I recommend not to take painkillers when trying for a baby. If you suffer from pain and need pain relief, acupuncture is very effective at relieving pain and doesn't have any negative side effects [171]. Alternatively, you can use topically applied gels or balms to relieve localised pain. In all cases, seek advice from your doctor.

Antidepressants

Research has shown the use of medications such as selective serotonin reuptake inhibitors (SSRIs) one month before conception can increase the risk of a baby developing a birth defect [172]. When taken during pregnancy, SSRIs can increase the risk of the baby being autistic or having a birth defect or speech/language disorder [173] [174] [175] [176] [177] [178] [179] [180] [181] [182].

If you have anxiety or depression, acupuncture and Chinese herbs are very effective at reducing these conditions without any side effects and can be safely continued throughout pregnancy [183]. Always consult with your doctor first.

Antiepileptic drugs

Antiepileptic drugs such as sodium valproate can cause birth defects and increase the risk of the child developing autism [184] [185] [186] [187]. Consult with your doctor about taking sodium valproate.

Statins

Medications such as statins can reduce levels of coenzyme Q10 within the body, which can reduce sperm and egg quality [332] [333] [334].

Improving your fertility checklist ☑

Here is a summary of things you can do to enhance your fertility:

☐ Be positive and use a vision board.

☐ Check your waist–hip ratio to see if your weight is correct.

☐ Don't diet; exercise if you need to lose weight.

☐ Don't have a bath after you ovulate; have a shower instead.

☐ Don't lift anything heavy.

☐ Don't smoke or take illegal drugs.

☐ Don't work night shifts.

☐ Drink no more than two glasses of red wine a week (125ml/1.4 units per glass).

☐ Exercise (cardio) two to three times a week plus soft exercises such as yoga, Pilates, t'ai chi and qi gong.

☐ Go to bed at around 10 p.m. and sleep for seven to eight hours.

☐ Have weekly acupuncture treatment and take Chinese herbs daily.

☐ Listen to your body; it knows best.

☐ Men should not sit down for more than a few hours at a time.

☐ Practise mindfulness or meditation.

☐ Reduce your exposure to air conditioning units.

☐ Reduce your exposure to air pollution or wear a mask.

☐ Reduce your exposure to chemicals and heavy metals.

☐ Reduce your exposure to negativity.

☐ Reduce your exposure to plastics.

☐ Reduce your stress by having fun.

☐ Reduce your use of painkillers, antidepressants, antiepileptic drugs and statins (always consult with your doctor first).

☐ Reduce your use of technology, i.e. mobile (cellular) phones, tablets, laptops (EMWs).

☐ Slow down your pace of life.

☐ Wear the right clothes and footwear for the season.

☐ Women should try to avoid giving blood.

Part Four

Optimising Your Diet

We've all heard the saying 'You are what you eat', but what does this mean in relation to fertility? For the Chinese, they see food not just as something to eat, but as a source of energy and as a medicine. Health and good fertility is the product of a sufficient accumulation and flow of energy in the body. Since food is seen as the major source of energy that we absorb every day, the proper selection of foods and timing of meals is an important method of manipulating energy for increasing your level of health and improving fertility.

Chapter 10

Chinese Dietary Therapy

For centuries the Chinese have added certain foods to their cooking to improve their health. Food is healthcare. Medicine isn't healthcare – its sick care. The Chinese believe that a happy stomach leads to a healthy body, because if the stomach is happy it will produce abundant amounts of energy and blood for the body's needs.

The stomach needs to be balanced at the right temperature for optimal digestion. For this reason, there is an old Chinese saying that 'You should chew your fluids and swallow your foods', which means that by chewing your fluids they become the same temperature as your body before they hit the stomach, to avoid damage from the cold; and if you swallow your food then it has been chewed enough so that the stomach can spend less energy processing it. A happy stomach is a happy body!

The Chinese avoid cold foods that can damage the stomach, such as ice, ice cream, salads, smoothies and other raw foods. This is why you never see salad on a menu in a Chinese restaurant. These foods are cold and uncooked, which makes the stomach work harder to process them, thereby weakening it. The opposite is also true: if the stomach becomes too hot it will spit stomach juices upwards like an erupting volcano causing heartburn (acid reflux). In such cases, the stomach needs to be cooled down by eating fewer hot, spicy, greasy foods and eating cooling foods such as mint and yoghurt.

Foods can be grouped into different natures: 'hot', 'cold', 'damp' or 'tonics'. Plants that take longer to grow, such as carrots, parsnips and cabbage, are more warming than those that grow quickly, such as lettuce, squash, radish and cucumber, which are cooling [188]. Tonics are foods that increase energy (qi) to promote general health and well-being and improve levels of leptin, which helps to improve hormone levels. Damp foods include dairy, cheese, cream, gluten and rich foods which make the digestive system work harder.

If a person has an imbalance, they can remedy this by eating the opposite food, for example cold (yin) foods for too much heat (yang) or hot (yang) foods for too much cold (yin). If a person has damp or is weak, tonic foods should be eaten. The aim of a good diet is to balance your yin and yang and boost your energy and blood levels. When they are all balanced and your energy levels are better, your body will be in a better position to become pregnant and maintain a healthy pregnancy.

The Chinese believe in eating like-for-like foods for their health problem. For example, eggs to improve egg quality (hen eggs, duck eggs, caviar, etc.) as well as red wine and beetroot juice to improve blood because it looks like blood.

Most people can use dietary therapy together with an optimised lifestyle and supplements to increase their fertility. For those men and women who are older or weaker, rectifying health with these measures can take longer. In such circumstances, Chinese herbs can be used to speed up the process of balancing yin and yang and boosting energy and blood levels.

Research has shown that women who were given dietary and lifestyle advice as well as coping mechanisms for dealing with their infertility had a marked improvement in pregnancy rates [189]. They became pregnant and lost weight too, had reduced anxiety and depression and improved self-esteem levels, all of which are important aspects of fertility treatment in Chinese medicine.

The Ideal Diet

Optimising your diet means not only eating good-quality foods for fertility but also eating regularly, when you're hungry and not on the go. You need to think about optimising every meal and every drink you have. Everything counts and is important in aiding your fertility:

- Avoid pre-made processed foods.
- Don't freeze meats or foods – cook and eat fresh.
- Don't microwave foods or drinks as they'll have little energy left in them and can also irritate the digestive tract, (see page 170).
- Eat foods that are organic.

All types of food are graded according to their quality. The quality of our food can affect our health and fertility. If you want good fertility then you need to nourish your body with good-quality food. People often choose the cheapest foods, thinking they look the same so they must be the same, but they are only the same skin-deep. Upon closer inspection, food varies greatly. For example, meat in one store can be very different to meat in another store. Non-organic meat contains a multitude of impurities that can damage both male and female fertility. You often get what you pay for, so paying a bit extra for better-quality food will greatly improve your health and chances of having a baby. You can't skimp on food if you want good health, as the saying goes: 'Pay the farmer now or the doctor later.'

A typical Western diet tends to be high in sugar and gluten, which are hard on the digestive system, making it weak and sluggish. These foods reduce the amount of energy and blood produced, making the body and fertility weaker. The ideal diet is a Paleo diet, one which we have evolved over millions of years to eat. A Paleo diet includes all foods in their natural form, as Nature intended, with nothing man-made – for example, bread, pasta, refined sugar, etc. Instead, we should eat fresh meat, fish, grains, fruit, vegetables and eat low glycaemic index (GI) carbohydrates like quinoa, oats, brown rice and sweet potatoes.

Most people eat with their eyes and their mouths rather than their stomachs. Any food that takes too long to digest, such as gluten, is bad for the stomach. Research has shown that people sensitive to gluten are more likely to be deficient in iron which can affect fertility [105]. In Chinese medicine, this is due to a weakened spleen not producing enough blood. For good health and fertility you should eat with both your mouth and your stomach. That way, the food you eat will be the best for your body and won't weaken it. It's no surprise that Chinese cuisine has evolved to be both good for the mouth and the stomach. Have you ever eaten a meal in a Chinese restaurant and then felt hungry again a few hours later? This is because it has been easy for the stomach to digest and has been processed efficiently. Learning what food is easy for your stomach to digest is a discovery process that can take time, but the rewards are great!

In recent years, there has been an explosion of coffee shops opening up. In Chinese medicine, stimulants such as caffeine in coffee are yang in nature and act as energy substitutes, helping to move blood. However, they can damage blood at the same time, while sugar in cakes, for example, acts as a replacement for a lack of blood (low blood sugar levels). Often women will crave sugar, especially when they are ovulating or have their period. If you crave coffee or cake, really your body needs more energy and blood; iron and ginseng can be taken instead. Coffee can reduce fertility so should be avoided when trying to fall pregnant [190] [191]. Dark chocolate (over 85 per cent cacao) is estimated to have only 1.7 per cent of the caffeine content of coffee, so that's still okay to eat!

Fertility clinics and nutritionists often recommend taking protein supplements to improve fertility, as protein is important in aiding follicle growth. Based upon my research, the ideal diet for fertility is a combination of protein, essential fatty acids, complex carbohydrates, vegetables high in iron and fruits rich in antioxidants. These are included in the diet plans outlined in Chapter Eleven.

Food Groups

There are 10 main food groups:

1. Carbohydrates.
2. Cold foods.
3. Fats.
4. Fibre.
5. Hot foods.
6. Proteins.
7. Sugars.
8. Tonics.
9. Vitamins and minerals.
10. Water.

Eating a balanced diet incorporating all these food groups is important for health and fertility. However, as we'll now discuss, some are more important than others.

Fats

We've all been told that fats are bad for our health, but, in fact, we all need some fats, just not too much and none of the bad ones. Bad fats are the trans-fatty acids (hydrogenated oils) found in processed foods and too much fat from red meat, all of which contain cholesterol. Our bodies need cholesterol to maintain good health; it helps to convert vitamin D in the skin, metabolises carbohydrates and is necessary for the production of male and female fertility hormones [192]. We just don't want too much of it – no more than 200mg/dL a day. Ideally our diet should contain no more than 10 per cent saturated fat in each day. As modern diets contain more red meat and processed foods, which contain trans-fatty acids, a lot of people can inadvertently overdose on bad fats, causing high cholesterol levels and infertility.

To reduce the effects of fats in our body, we can increase our consumption of lipotropics. Lipotropics increase the liver's production of lecithin, which keeps cholesterol levels down. Lipotropics include methionine, choline, inositol and betaine and are found in a wide range of foods, such as Brazil nuts, turkey, chicken, eggs, yogurt, etc. Be careful when selecting foods that proclaim they are either low in fat or fat-free as often manufacturers have replaced the tasty fats with something even worse for our health – refined sugar!

Sugar

Sugar is the new bad kid on the block, when once it was fats. Naturally-occurring sugars, for example those found in fruit, are actually good for the body and help to fuel muscles, nerves and the brain. It's the refined form of sugar that is the problem. A lot of people crave refined sugars, which are found in food such as cakes, biscuits, sweets (candy) and fizzy drinks. Craving sugar is like an addiction and acts on the brain in the same way as cocaine [193]. Refined sugar passes quickly into the bloodstream in large amounts, giving the stomach and pancreas a shock. The digestive system is then weakened and food cannot be digested properly. This leads to a blood sugar imbalance and further cravings for sugar.

If you crave refined sugar, your body is most likely tired and deficient and wants quick energy. Instead of giving it sugar, have a nap, reduce your energy expenditure, eat more protein- and iron-rich foods and take ginseng and iron supplements (see pages 190 and 191). The body would rather have more energy than more sugar. Eating too much sugar can create heat (excessive yang) and deplete yin levels, thereby damaging fertility. Eating a diet that's high in refined, processed sugar will also affect insulin levels. High levels of insulin can increase levels of testosterone in the body causing polycystic ovary syndrome (PCOS). New research has shown that eating too much sugar affects the uterus lining, making it inhospitable to an embryo trying to implant into the uterus wall [1].

Essential fatty acids

Essential fatty acids (EFAs) are a group of oils known as long-chain polyunsaturated fatty acids (PUFAs). They come in two types: omega-3 (linolenic acid) and omega-6 (linoleic acid). Omega-9 is not considered an essential fatty acid as our bodies can make it from omega-3 or -6. Our bodies cannot produce omega-3 or -6, so we have to get them through our diet.

Modern Western diets tend to overdose on omega-6 and under consume omega-3. Research has shown that men who have more omega-6 than -3 in their body have reduced sperm quality [194]. Omega-6 is mainly found in vegetable oils such as sunflower and corn oils, while the highest amount of omega-3 is found in certain types of fish, seeds and dark greens, such as:

- anchovies
- butterfish
- cereal grasses (rice, rye, oats, maize, buckwheat, millet)
- chard
- chia seed
- flaxseed
- hempseed
- herring
- kale
- parsley
- pilchard
- pumpkin seed
- rainbow trout
- rapeseed
- salmon
- sardines
- walnuts

Prolonged stress, such as anxiety or dieting, can put the body into a state of resistance – level 2 of the body's stress response (see page 137) – causing a reduction in lipid reserves. Lipids are an organic compound made up of fats and oils that are important for bodily functions and for fertility. As most people are stressed for more than two hours, which is the time needed to put the body into the resistance phase, most people are deficient in lipids and EFAs (omega-3). Additionally, poor lifestyle habits can also affect the metabolism of omega-3 in the body, worsening fertility. These include:

- a deficiency of vitamin B_6, zinc and magnesium
- dieting
- excessive consumption of alcohol, trans-fatty acids, sugar or animal fat
- exposure to pollutants
- smoking

Women with a deficiency of PUFAs (omega-3 and -6) in their diet may have a heightened immune system which can prevent implantation of the embryo into the uterus wall. Research has shown that olive oil, which is high in omega-3 and -6, can regulate important immune messengers called cytokines, especially TH1, which when reduced allows a fertilised embryo to implant [138].

PUFAs such as omega-3 are important for good fertility. They contain antioxidants, such as vitamin E, which are needed to balance the level of free radicals in the body that can damage eggs and sperm, and prevent implantation. EFAs are used as an energy source during maturation of the egg and during the period it moves down the fallopian tube before implanting into the uterus wall.

EFAs are particularly important during pregnancy, as they are required for the development of the baby's brain and eyes. The recommended daily intake of essential fatty acids is 14g. One tablespoon of flaxseed oil a day, for example, has a total EFA of 8.9g.

Protein

Protein is important in building up good levels of fertility, especially in men or women who don't eat a lot of red meat or who are vegetarian. A deficiency of protein can manifest as weak muscles, nails, hair loss, slow healing, general lack of energy and strength, poor concentration and emotional stability, persistent infections and allergies.

Some fertility clinics recommend drinking large quantities of milk daily for protein. However, drinking large quantities of milk every day will damage the digestive system, which will damage fertility. Below is a list of foods that contain more protein that milk – 15g of protein per 100g serving – that won't damage your digestive system. Protein from red meat sources can reduce fertility so these have been excluded here.

- Halibut 23g
- Parmesan 32g
- Tuna steak (light) 32g
- Pumpkin seeds 30g
- Turkey (organic) 30g
- Peanuts 25-28g
- Edam cheese 27g
- Tilapia 26g
- Canned tuna (light) 25g
- Cheddar cheese 25g
- Seitan 25g
- Chicken (organic) 31g
- Salmon 24g
- Almonds 21g
- Sardines 21g
- Cod 20g
- Mackerel 20g
- Pistachios 20g
- Tempeh 20g
- Pollock 19g
- Cashew nuts 18g
- Mozzarella 18g
- Chia seeds 17g
- Walnuts 15-17g

Factors that can deplete protein include:
- poor diet, refined sugars, alcohol and coffee
- stress, worry, overworking and trauma

Red meat

Red meat is good for your health and fertility. It is a rich source of protein, iron, zinc and vitamin B_{12}. We need to have some of it in our diet, but not too much. Excessive red meat consumption can be bad for health and fertility. In the United States, anabolic sex steroid hormones are administered to cattle and other animals for growth promotion 60–90 days before slaughter [195]. This practice was banned in Europe in the 1980s. Processed red meats have previously been shown to have higher concentrations of hormone residues compared with other meats raising concerns regarding the potential reproductive health consequences of consuming these foods.

The best red meat to eat is organic lean red meat that hasn't been frozen or processed; as close to Nature as it can be and only one serving a week. Research has shown that eating too much non-organic red meat can damage male fertility as red meat is high in saturated fat and low in EFAs [195]. Men should reduce their red meat intake and replace it with fish and algae (spirulina and chlorella) to improve their semen quality.

Protein shakes

Eating a lot of protein is important in helping fertility as it aids follicle growth as well as helps to maintaining a pregnancy. I recommend taking protein supplements in between meals, for example one protein shake before lunch and another before dinner, when trying for a baby. A good protein supplement to take is organic whey protein, which is available from most health food stores.

Carbohydrates

There are two main types of carbohydrates: simple and complex. Simple carbohydrates include white and brown sugar, glucose, corn syrups and fruit juices, etc, which are bad. Complex carbohydrates include whole grains, yams, brown rice, potatoes, carrots, broccoli and green beans, etc.

Complex carbohydrates contain a monosaccharide called sialic acid, which is important in the growth of the egg, its maturation, ovulation and subsequent fertilisation [133]. Adequate levels of complex carbohydrates are needed for the hormone FSH to interact with the follicles, making them grow [134]. It's therefore important for egg quality and fertility to make sure that the woman eats plenty of complex carbohydrates, around 250–350g per day.

Vegetarianism

More and more people are choosing to become vegetarian, especially with animal welfare being so poor and the inclusion of antibiotics and steroids in meat. However, being a vegetarian is not easy. It requires a varied diet to ensure all minerals and vitamins are included. Most vegetarians do not eat a varied diet and become weak, and iron- and protein-deficient, leading to poor fertility. From a Chinese medicine point of view, most vegetarians have a lack of blood and yang. Vegetarians tend to have lower levels of testosterone and vitamin B_{12}. This can affect both male and female fertility.

If you are vegetarian, you need to be very diligent with your diet and eat a wide range of good-quality foods to maintain high levels of energy and blood as well as eat enough protein and omega-3 from non-animal sources. With today's hectic lifestyle this is a challenge and can lead to a lack of blood. Half of women in India, where a high percentage of the population is vegetarian, are anaemic [196].

Veganism is also on the rise, with concerns around climate change, animal welfare and health compelling more and more people to follow a plant-based way of life. However, vegans can have more exaggerated symptoms than vegetarians. Vegans often have lower levels of DHEA [343]. Higher levels of DHEA are better for egg growth. They also have higher levels of SHBG, which reduces testosterone levels and affects egg growth [344] [345]. Vegetarians and vegans tend to be deficient in iodine [197]. On the plus side, vegetarians and vegans tend to have lower levels of mercury because they don't eat fish, which is good for their fertility.

Caffeine

Caffeine is similar to sugar – it's a stimulant with side effects. Caffeine helps to move blood, giving us a false sense of having more energy, but it also damages blood at the same time. Both coffee and tea contains caffeine. Caffeine can increase levels of SHBG, which reduce free testosterone levels needed for egg and sperm development [346].

Men tend to drink more coffee than women [198], but research has shown that coffee can damage the DNA housed in the sperm's head [199] [191]. Women trying to fall pregnant should not consume caffeine as it depletes the absorption of calcium which is needed to activate the egg at the time of fertilisation [200]. Research has also shown that caffeine can delay the time it takes for a woman to fall pregnant [190]. Decaf coffee is better, but there can still be traces of caffeine present.

If you crave coffee, then your body really needs more energy. Try replacing coffee with either ginseng if you're tired and replace sugar with leafy greens and take an iron supplement (see page 191).

Alcohol

I often get asked if people can still drink alcohol when trying for a baby. I believe that having a couple of glasses of red wine (125ml/1.4 units per glass) a week can be of benefit to fertility, but no more than that. Red wine helps the blood to move. It also aids in relaxation and fun, which can be of great benefit when trying for a baby, since most couples are stressed. By still drinking some alcohol, you can avoid being put in awkward situations with friends when they ask why you aren't drinking. I would say red wine is okay, as it mimics the colour of blood, which forms part of Chinese dietary therapy, eating like-for-like (see page 157). Spirits tend to be very yang in nature and beer/lager heavy on the digestion, hence why I recommend red wine only. Unfortunately, white wine doesn't have the same positive effects upon the blood as red wine, so I don't recommend drinking it.

Women should be careful not to drink too much alcohol as it can reduce their fertility [201]. Men should also be careful not to drink too much alcohol, which can increase the amount of heat in their body and damage sperm production and sperm DNA. More than 5–25 units of alcohol a week has been shown to significantly reduce fertility in men [202] [203]. Too much alcohol reduces testosterone levels, which are important in both male and female fertility, although more so in men. Excessive alcohol intake causes increased levels of oestrogens in males as well as a loss of libido, an enlarged prostate and fatigue [69]. Excessive amounts of alcohol also affect the pituitary gland and its release of fertility hormones in males [69].

Water

Being adequately hydrated is very important. Water makes up 55–60 per cent of the body. A good amount of water ensures blood moves smoothly and tissues are nourished. I recommend drinking 2 litres (½ gallon) of water a day. It sounds like a lot and drinking this much water a day can take practise and time. If you work at a desk, put a two-litre glass or metal bottle on it and sip from it throughout the day. You will then achieve your daily quota.

Initially you'll probably find that you'll be going to the toilet more often until your body gets used to the increase in fluids. You may also find that as you drink more, you feel more thirsty. This is because the body believes it has come to an oasis after a prolonged drought and wants to stock up on fluids. Don't drink water straight from the tap; filter it first to remove any traces of chemicals and medications that can affect your health and fertility. Drink water from a glass or porcelain cup rather than from plastic.

Hot foods

Hot foods can be divided into two types: warm or hot. Warm foods include onion, garlic, ginger, wasabi, paprika and turmeric. These foods are often good for the digestion as they help to keep the stomach warm.

The stomach needs to be warm to facilitate the breakdown of foods and digestion. Hot foods include chilli. Eating chilli can create internal heat in the body, damaging bodily fluids such as cervical mucus and semen. There is an old wives' tale from India that says: 'If a man wants to have children, he should stop eating chilli.' I would recommend that men don't eat chilli at all. Women can eat chilli if they feel very cold.

Cold foods

Cold foods include salads, ice, ice cream and chilled water and foods. Salads are seen in the West as being healthy and good for you as they are natural and low in calories. However, salads are cold and raw which makes the stomach work harder to process them. This makes the stomach weaker, which affects digestion and reduces the production of energy and blood. Cold and raw foods also damage yang [188]. Ice and ice cream do the same thing – they make the stomach cold and inefficient. The stomach likes to be warm, hence why foods such as ginger are good for it.

Another food trend at the moment is the drinking of raw juices. Raw juices can stress the stomach in the same way as salads, weakening it and causing a yang deficiency. Having a warm liquid ginseng drink in the morning would be better for your digestion, energy levels and fertility.

Tonics

Tonics are foods that can boost and aid your digestive system. When your digestive system is working more efficiently, your energy levels will be better. A good example of a tonic food is ginseng. Ginseng gives you more energy and can uplift the digestive system, thereby aiding metabolism and the production of blood needed for the body. It can also regulate leptin levels, which regulates fertility hormones [204] and can also increase levels of TH2, which protects an embryo implanting into the uterus lining [336]. Another example of a tonic is probiotics. Probiotics increase good bacteria in the stomach, which improves stomach function, digestion and cognitive function [205].

Microwaves

Microwaves have become the norm for most people in today's world because they are quick and convenient. However, research has shown that foods heated in microwaves can contain harmful chemicals which have leached into the food from the plastic container [206] [207].

I believe that food that has been heated using a microwave offers little energetic value. Its energy has been zapped and it lacks vitality. Essentially, it's dead food. Eating microwaved food regularly can lead to a lack of energy, tiredness and a weakened stomach as the heat from the microwaved food can irritate and damage the digestive tract [208] [209].

Microwaves work by making the atoms in the food rub together to generate heat, which cooks the food. However, as you're eating the food, the atoms are still vibrating, which will affect the cells in the body that they come into contact with. You can normally tell when food has been microwaved to heat it up as your stomach is unusually hot after eating a microwaved meal. I recommend avoiding microwaved food or fluids whenever possible and always cook from fresh.

Foods That Affect Oestrogen Levels

There are many plants that contain naturally occurring oestrogen within them. These plants are called phytoestrogens. When we eat these plants, we can disrupt the normal level of oestrogens within our body. Combined with man-made oestrogens means most people have irregular oestrogen levels. Having too much oestrogen can affect male and female fertility. There are three types of phytoestrogens. Each has a different bonding strength with oestrogen receptors within our body:

1. Coumestans.

2. Flavonoids

3. Lignans

Asians and vegetarians tend to have high levels of phytoestrogens in their bodies because of dietary choices[210], which can be a problem for fertility. Both men and women should limit their intake of phytoestrogens. Women should avoid foods that contain soya as it can interfere with ovulation.

Coumestans

Coumestans are a group of phytoestrogens that have a weak effect upon oestrogen levels in the body. Foods containing coumestans include split peas, pinto beans, lima beans, alfalfa and clover. I would avoid eating clover as it may cause infertility in females[211].

Flavonoids

Flavonoids are classified into six classes: flavonols, flavones, flavanols, flavanonols, flavanones and isoflavones. Isoflavones are the most widely eaten type of flavonoid. Isoflavones (including genistein) can have a negative effect upon female fertility[210].

All phytoestrogens can bind to oestrogen receptors (ESR1 and ESR2) making them inactive, but especially isoflavones[210]. This can have a negative effect upon female fertility by affecting the menstrual cycle and the thickness of the uterus lining, which can then affect implantation. Foods that contain isoflavones include: berries, wine, grains, nuts and other legumes such as chickpeas, peas, peanuts, alfalfa, mung beans and especially clover[210].

Genistein is found exclusively in soya foods, such as soya milk, tofu, miso and tempeh[191]. Unknown to a lot of people, soya is found in meat substitute products, energy bars, sports drinks, imitation dairy products, some cereals, bread, biscuits, vitamin supplements, chocolate spreads, ice cream, cheeses and infant products, making it important to always read food labels [210]. The Japanese consume the highest amount of soya foods in the world and also have the highest use of in-vitro fertilisation (IVF) in the world [212] [213]. Soya products can reduce the LH surge needed to mature the egg and reduce the effectiveness of FSH upon the ovary [214]. Currently, there are no known side effects of soya consumption in males [215].

Lignans

Lignans are one of the important phytoestrogens obtained from dietary sources. Lignans mimic oestrogen and weakly bind to oestrogen receptors, thus preventing some actions of oestrogen. Foods that contain lignans include: sesame seeds, sunflower seeds, cashew nuts, tofu, kale, chocolate, pears, raisins, kiwi, grapefruit, oranges, broccoli, white cabbage, carrots, strawberries, peaches, Brussels sprouts, apricots and especially flaxseed [191]. Lignans have a limited impact upon male and female fertility.

Foods That Affect Progesterone Levels

Foods that contain apigenin can increase levels of progesterone [216] [217], which can help to maintain the uterus lining and aid implantation. Apigenin is in higher levels in chamomile tea, celery, yarrow, tarragon, liquorice, flax, passionflower, spearmint, basil and oregano [218]. It is best to eat these foods once you've ovulated and not before as once progesterone levels become high, they switch off the production of GnRH from the hypothalamus, which can prevent follicle growth.

Foods that can block progesterone contain the compounds chlorophylline (green vegetables), hesperetin (lemons, oranges, grapefruit, tangerines and peppermint), homocysteine and a-tocopherol (vitamin E) [219] [220]. As good fertility and pregnancy relies on adequate levels of progesterone, it's best to not eat these foods once you've ovulated.

Foods That Affect Testosterone Levels

There are several groups of foods that can affect testosterone levels. For men it can be of benefit to increase testosterone levels, while for women with obese-type PCOS, it's best to reduce testosterone levels.

Foods that contain the compounds beta-carotene (apricots, sweet potatoes, broccoli, pumpkin, carrots, mangoes and peaches), chlorophylline (green vegetables), chlorogenic acid (coffee and black tea), homocysteine, taxifolin (red onions, milk thistle) and a-tocopherol have been shown in research to block dihydrotestosterone (DHT) [219], which is bad for fertility, especially in men. DHT is made through the conversion of testosterone. High levels of DHT in men are associated with a good sperm count and motility [221]. The plant *tribulus terrestris* can increase DHT levels and improve male fertility [221].

Foods that can increase testosterone levels are the same as for progesterone above. Apigenin affects the Leydig cells, which produce testosterone [222]. Eating foods with apigenin is good for women with low anti-Müllerian hormone (AMH) levels or men with poor sperm quality. Vegetarians should make sure they eat plenty of foods that contain apigenin.

Chapter 11

Female and Male Diet Plans

The following diet plans are based on the information outlined in the previous chapter, in order to maximise your hormones and fertility.

Foods should be fresh, not frozen, and lightly cooked using a traditional cooker or steamer – no microwaves please. When cooking vegetables, it's best to steam them until they are crunchy not soft and use a gas or electric hob to cook meats. No wood burning stoves or BBQs as the smoke from these can reduce anti-Müllerian hormone (AMH) levels.

Normally, it would be beneficial to include foods that contain oestrogen for the first part of your menstrual cycle and foods that increase progesterone levels in the second part of your cycle. However, due to the exposure of man-made chemicals in our daily lives, most people have irregular levels of oestrogens, which can cause male and female infertility. Therefore, my diet plans aim to regulate and reduce oestrogen levels rather than boost them. This is especially important if you decide to move onto IVF at a later stage, as during IVF treatment, oestrogen levels rise dramatically to around 15,000 pmol/L (4,000 pg/mL), which can contribute to the development of oestrogen type cancers (breast, uterus and ovaries) [3].

There are foods that are good for blood, yin and jing for the first part of your menstrual cycle, before you ovulate, and foods that can enhance progesterone and are good for yang in the second part of your cycle once you've ovulated. By eating foods that affect not only yin and yang but also oestrogen and progesterone, you can maximise the effects of your diet on your hormones and fertility. For male fertility, it's best to reduce oestrogen levels as they can affect testosterone levels and sperm quality.

If you feel cold, add spices such as paprika or ginger to your dishes to warm you up. If, however, you get heartburn (acid reflux) then remove these spices as heartburn indicates that they are too hot for your stomach.

Protein should be sourced from plants rather than meats as overconsumption of these is associated with infertility, especially in men. Men should replace red meat with fish and algae, such as spirulina and chlorella. Women should avoid algae as it can affect implantation. If you need to eat red meat, then it should be organic and fresh, not from frozen and no more than once a week. Vegetables should be organic if possible. Citrus fruits contain both hesperetin, apigenin, sugars and are simple carbohydrates, which affect levels of progesterone and implantation. It's therefore best not to drink any citrus fruit juices.

Try not to take any nonsteroidal anti-inflammatory drugs (NSAIDs), such as diclofenac, naproxen and etoricoxib, as all three can reduce progesterone levels [223]. For those trying for their next child, the woman should take extra omega-3 supplements (not from cod liver oil). For those with a low AMH level, take bee pollen, royal jelly, myo-inositol, coenzyme Q10 and DHEA daily (see Chapter Seven), as they can improve egg quality. Those who are tired can take maca or ginseng. All women and men should take a good-quality prenatal supplement (see Chapter Twelve).

The Female Diet Plan

Pre-ovulation: from day 1 of your menstrual cycle

This diet plan starts from the first day of your menstrual bleed until you ovulate. It's designed to regulate oestrogen levels and boost energy, yin, jing, omega-3 and blood levels, thereby improving egg quality and ovulation. It's set out in a menu style for you to pick various breakfast, lunch or dinner options together with specific snacks and drinks, as well as supplements.

Drink options

- Coffee lovers who need a lift in the morning can have one cup of decaf coffee, but remember that decaf coffee still has some caffeine in it. If you can, avoid coffee as it reduces your body's ability to absorb calcium and causes irregular levels of SHBG. Try a ginseng or maca drink instead.

- Tea lovers need to be careful too, as a lot of tea contains caffeine and tannin, which can affect the absorption of calcium and iron. Different teas have different effects. Black (English) tea is warming and, like coffee, it contains chlorogenic acid, which can affect levels of dihydrotestosterone (DHT) and sperm quality. One cup of decaf black tea in the morning is okay. If you feel too warm or have heartburn, don't drink black tea. Instead, drink mint, peppermint or green tea (decaf) as these will cool you down.

- Ideal hot drinks that aid the stomach and health are hot water with peppermint or ginger. If you have heartburn, omit the ginger. Other hot drinks you can have include rooibos tea, herbal teas, hot water with lemon and hot cacao with or without ginger.

- Cold drinks include water, water with a slice of lemon or orange or beetroot juice by itself. None of these cold drinks should be chilled or have ice in – serve them at room temperature only.

- Try to drink plenty of water. It should not be chilled – serve it at either room temperature or warm. Two litres (½ gallon) of water a day is ideal. Do not refill plastic bottles. Instead, use a new plastic bottle, or a glass or porcelain cup. (See 'Know your plastics' on page 143 for more on this.)

Supplements

- A good-quality prenatal supplement.
- Iron: 20mg (even though it's already in the prenatal supplement).
- Royal jelly or bee pollen.

Snack options

- Apples, apricots, cherries, dates, figs, grapes.
- Almonds, cashew nuts, sesame seeds, sunflower seeds, walnuts.
- Boiled eggs.
- Oat bars.
- Sushi (fish) with wasabi.

Breakfast options

- Eggs (scrambled, poached or boiled) with salmon and mashed avocado with either lemon and olive oil or a pinch of paprika if you feel cold.
- Wheat-free cereal with almond or rice milk. Try to avoid cow's milk as it's too heavy on the digestive system, which can weaken the body, and contains oestrogen. Avoid soya milk completely.
- Poached eggs with asparagus.
- Oats with nuts and seeds with either almond or rice milk.
- Omelette with spinach and/or potato.
- Salmon with parsley, poached eggs and asparagus.
- Herring and egg salad.

Lunch options

- Jacket potato with sardines, mackerel or eggs.
- Sweet potato with choice of fillings above.

- Soups are ideal in cold seasons: chicken, fish or beetroot, tomato and lentil soup.
- Sushi (fish) with seaweed and wasabi.
- Mixed bean (kidney, black and aduki) salad.
- Chicken with steamed asparagus and baby potatoes.
- Sardines with tomato, garlic, chickpea and feta cheese salad with a lemon juice dressing.

Dinner options

- Mussels with coconut milk and lemongrass.
- Salmon with steamed kelp and brown rice.
- Clam linguine (wheat free) with almonds.
- Trout stuffed with lemon and parsley with baby potatoes and green beans.
- Lentils either baked with aubergine or as a lasagne.
- Cod with steamed kale and brown rice.
- Sea bass with ginger and spring onions.
- Steak with a spinach, walnut and feta cheese salad and sweet potato fries.
- Lamb with apricots and squash casserole.

Post-ovulation: from ovulation until the end of your cycle

This diet plan starts from when you ovulate until the end of your menstrual cycle. It's designed to boost progesterone and yang levels, thereby improving implantation and pregnancy.

Drink options

- Coffee lovers who need a lift in the morning can have one cup of decaf. Otherwise, if you can, avoid coffee altogether and have a ginseng or maca drink instead.
- Chamomile tea is ideal. One to two cups of black (English) or green tea (decaf) is also fine. If you feel too warm or have

heartburn, don't drink black tea. Instead have decaf green tea. No peppermint tea now as it can block progesterone. Other hot drinks you can have include rooibos tea, spearmint tea, hot water with ginger, ginseng, herbal teas and hot cacao with ginger. Ideal hot drinks that aid the stomach and health are hot water with ginger. If you have heartburn, omit the ginger.

- Cold drinks include water or beetroot juice. Cold drinks should not be chilled or have ice in them – serve them at room temperature only. No lemons, oranges, grapefruit, tangerines once you've ovulated as these contain hesperetin, which can block progesterone.
- Try to drink plenty of water, either at room temperature or warm. Two litres (½ gallon) a day is ideal.

Supplements

- A good-quality prenatal supplement.
- Iron: 20mg (even though it's already in the prenatal supplement).
- Royal jelly or bee pollen.

Snack options

- Celery sticks.
- Cherries, dates and raspberries.
- Chestnuts, pistachio nuts, sunflower seeds, sesame seeds and walnuts.

Breakfast options

- Eggs (scrambled, poached or boiled) with salmon and mashed avocado with olive oil and a touch of paprika.
- Wheat-free cereal with either almond or rice milk; try to avoid cow's milk. Avoid soya milk completely.
- Oats with nuts, seeds and flaxseed.
- Spelt bread with raspberry jam.

- Soft-boiled eggs with anchovies and parsley.

Lunch options

- Prawn salad with Tabasco or cayenne pepper and parsley.
- Quinoa with salmon or apricots and pistachios.
- Pasta (wheat free) with anchovies, crushed red peppers and either yarrow or tarragon.
- Sweet potato soup.
- Baked sweet potato with spinach and chickpeas.
- Butternut squash soup.

Dinner options

- Buckwheat (soba) noodles with coconut sauce (no soya), sesame seeds, cucumber and ginger.
- Prawns with tomatoes, garlic and brown rice.
- Anchovies with lamb and rosemary.
- Lamb with sweet potato and spice curry.
- Salmon with mustard seeds and a lentil salad.
- Spaghetti with olive oil, basil and oregano sauce.
- Mussels with coconut milk, cloves, lemongrass and coriander.

The Male Diet Plan

The male diet plan is designed for better semen quality with foods that improve testosterone, increase antioxidants and harmonise yang levels.

Most men love red meat. However, red meat can damage male fertility. It is therefore best to reduce red meat consumption. I would recommend one serving of red meat and two servings of white meat a week. Both should be organic and not from frozen. Research has shown that replacing meat with fish improves sperm count and morphology [195]. White fish (such as cod, haddock, sea bass, pollack, coley, hake, whiting, plaice, sole, John Dory, halibut, flounder and turbot) improves sperm morphology, while dark fish (such as sardines, herring, anchovies, salmon and trout) improves sperm count. Consuming two servings of fish a week in lieu of two servings of processed red meat a week was associated with a 60 per cent higher total normal sperm count [195]. There are also other better sources of protein than meat, and without the side effects, for example algae (spirulina and chlorella-see Chapter Twelve).

Drink options

- One cup of either decaf coffee or decaf tea. Sorry guys, but caffeine is bad for sperm DNA!
- Mint, peppermint, chamomile, chrysanthemum (ju hua), dandelion, elderflower, ginger or green tea (decaf). If you have heartburn, omit ginger. Other hot drinks include rooibos tea, herbal teas and hot water with a slice of lemon.
- Cold drinks include water and beetroot juice. Cold drinks should not be chilled or have ice – serve them at room temperature only.
- Drink plenty of water – not chilled, but either at room temperature or warm. Two litres (½ gallon) a day is ideal.

Supplements

- Coenzyme q10 (600mg).
- Essential fatty acids (omega-3) (14g).
- L-arginine (15g).
- Lycopene (5-10mg).
- Selenium (200mcg).
- Spirulina or chlorella (5g).
- Vitamin C (1g) [136].
- Vitamin E (100-400mg) [224] [225].
- Zinc (15mg).

Snack options

- Apples, blueberries, cranberries, figs, grapefruit, melon, pears, pineapple, plums and watermelon.
- Almonds, pistachio nuts, pumpkin seeds, sunflower seeds and walnuts.
- Celery sticks.
- Protein bars or shakes.

Breakfast options

- Eggs (scrambled, poached or boiled) with salmon and mashed avocado with either lemon or olive oil.
- Pilchards with eggs, chopped tomatoes and parsley.
- Sardines with eggs and parsley.
- Wheat-free cereal with either almond or rice milk. No cow's milk as it has oestrogens in it.
- Poached eggs with asparagus.
- Oats with nuts and seeds.
- Grapefruit.
- Mixed fruit (see 'Snack options' above) with natural yoghurt.

Lunch options

- Prawn salad with Tabasco or cayenne pepper and parsley.
- Quinoa with salmon or apricots and pistachios.
- Grilled chicken with a spinach and kidney bean salad.
- Jacket potato with tuna and sweetcorn.
- Sushi (fish) with seaweed.
- Pasta (wheat free) with anchovies, crushed red peppers and either yarrow or tarragon.
- Herring and egg salad.
- Chicken with steamed asparagus and baby potatoes.

Dinner options

- Prawns with tomatoes, garlic and rice.
- Anchovies with lamb and rosemary.
- Trout stuffed with lemon and parsley with baby potatoes and green beans.
- Clams with linguine (wheat free) and almonds.
- Octopus salad with potato and green beans.
- Rainbow trout with lemon, dill and thyme.
- Lamb and cumin burger with steamed spinach and parsnip chips.
- Pasta (wheat free) with garlic, anchovies, capers and red peppers.
- Salmon with mustard seeds and a lentil salad.
- Mussels with coconut milk, cloves, lemongrass and coriander (no chilli).
- Steak with a spinach, walnut and feta cheese salad and sweet potato fries.
- Anchovies with lamb and rosemary.

Optimising your diet checklist ☑

☐ Avoid drinking liquids out of plastic containers.

☐ Avoid foods in plastics.

☐ Avoid frozen foods.

☐ Avoid chilled sandwiches, salads and ice cream.

☐ Both men and women should take a good-quality prenatal supplement daily.

☐ Cut out or reduce caffeine.

☐ Cut out refined sugar.

☐ Don't eat on the go or when working.

☐ Don't use microwaves.

☐ Drink no more than two glasses of red wine (125ml/1.4 units per glass) a week.

☐ Drink 2 litres (½ gallon) of water a day.

☐ Eat freshly made foods.

☐ Eat only when hungry.

☐ Men should cut out chilli.

☐ Men should substitute red meat for fish and algae.

☐ Women should avoid taking algae supplements.

Chapter 12

Supplements

There are many supplements that can enhance male and female fertility. I've done my own extensive research into the fertility benefits of various supplements and have listed them below. The daily dosage is the total daily amount, which includes sources from both food and supplements. Please check the dosage carefully as different supplements have greatly different dose ranges.

Most prenatal supplements will contain the vitamin and minerals listed below, but not necessarily in the same quantity. People with different types of infertility will need different vitamins and minerals at varying dosage levels. If in doubt, consult a nutritionist that specialises in fertility.

Dosages

A milligram (mg) is one thousandth of 1 gram, while a microgram (mcg) is one millionth of 1 gram. Therefore, 1g equals 1000mg or 1,000,000mcg, while 1mg equals 1000mcg.

Agnus castus is also called vitex agnus castus or 'chaste tree', which refers to its ability to decrease sexual desire and promote chastity in women [226]. It can help to reduce PMS and regulate the menstrual cycle [227] [226] [228] [229]. It has the most benefit when a woman has an irregular menstrual cycle (oligomenorrhoea) [230]. I recommend a daily dose of 10–15 drops from a tincture.

Alpha lipoic acid (ALA) is also known as thioctic acid. It's present in the body in small quantities where it reacts with B group vitamins to speed up metabolic reactions needed for energy production. It's a powerful antioxidant that enhances other antioxidants such as vitamins C and E. I recommend a daily dose of 50–100mg.

Bee pollen is a rich source of protein, essential fatty acids and vitamin B_{12} and is considered one of Nature's most completely nourishing foods for people [231]. In Chinese medicine, it is used to enhance jing, yin and blood levels. I recommend a daily dose of 2–5g.

Beta-carotene is converted into vitamin A only when the body needs it [191]. It is an antioxidant and can help to prevent damage caused by free radicals [224] [232]. Do not take if you have hypothyroidism (underactive thyroid) as levels will already be high [233]. Beta-carotene can be found in apricots, sweet potatoes, broccoli, pumpkin, carrots, mangoes and peaches. I recommend a daily dose of 3–6mg. Men should reduce their intake of this compound in their diet as it can reduce testosterone levels, which can affect sperm production [219].

Biotin is essential in the synthesis and metabolism of glucose, fatty acids, amino acids and stress hormones. As biotin has the potential to improve glucose metabolism by stimulating insulin release, it can be of benefit to women with polycystic ovary syndrome (PCOS), who are often insulin resistant. Biotin is found in meat, oily fish, whole grains, rice, nuts, cauliflower and egg yolk. I recommend a daily dose of 30mcg.

Bromelain is found in the stem of pineapples. It has anti-inflammatory properties and has been found to be a useful treatment for inflammatory infertility problems such as endometriosis [234] [235]. However, it acts to decrease levels of prostaglandins E2, which are necessary for ovulation and implantation [168] [236]. Prostaglandins E2 are needed for successful implantation of the embryo into the uterus wall [354] [355]. I therefore don't recommend taking bromelain supplements or eating pineapple stems unless you have endometriosis, in which case I recommend a daily dose of 500–1000mg.

Calcium is important for our bones. Around 99 per cent of the calcium we consume goes into our bones and teeth [231]. Calcium is also needed to activate the egg at the time of fertilisation [200]. It plays an important role in blood clotting and the production of energy. Calcium is absorbed in the small intestine, which is dependent upon vitamin D. Calcium is found in dairy products, eggs, broccoli, tinned salmon, nuts and seeds. I would recommend not sourcing calcium from dairy products as dairy can weaken the digestive system, which weakens the body and fertility. There is more absorbable calcium in vegetables such as broccoli than there is in milk [231]. Caffeine affects the absorption of calcium. I recommend a daily dose of 1000mg.

Chlorella, also known as blue algae (*chlorellaceae*), is similar to spirulina. It helps to tonify the essence (jing) and is ideal for sperm quality. It contains vitamins B, C and E as well as zinc and iron. As it can boost the immune system (TH1 cells), much like spirulina, it can affect implantation of the embryo into the uterus wall [237]. For this reason, I would recommend that only men take this supplement. I recommend a daily dose of 5g.

Choline is vital for the development of your baby's memory in future life. It becomes depleted during pregnancy and lactation. Egg yolks and green leafy vegetables are a good source of choline. I recommend a daily dose of 450mg.

Chromium deficiency is thought to be common and linked to glucose intolerance, weight gain, depression, infertility and a decreased sperm count [238]. Chromium is found in egg yolks, red meat, cheese, fruit, whole grains, honey, vegetables, black pepper and thyme. I recommend a daily dose of 100mcg.

Cod liver oil contains important omega-3s and vitamin A. However, as the level of vitamin A within cod liver oil is difficult to determine, it's easy to overdose, which can lead to birth defects [239]. I would therefore recommend women avoid cod liver oil supplements when trying to conceive and take beta-carotene instead. Men can continue to take cod liver oil supplements when trying to conceive. I recommend a daily dose of 1000mg.

Coenzyme Q10 is a vitamin-like substance that processes oxygen in cells and generates energy-rich molecules. It is vital in male fertility when the man suffers from poor sperm motility [224] [240]. Levels of coenzyme Q10 decrease from the age of 30. Medications such as statins can also reduce levels of coenzyme Q10 within the body [332] [333] [334]. Females who took coenzyme Q10 had improved egg quality [241]. It's been shown to help antral follicle count (AFC) when taken together with DHEA at a daily dose of 600mg and DHEA at 25mg [32]. Coenzyme Q10 is found in meat, fish, eggs, whole grains, nuts and green vegetables. I recommend a daily dose of 600mg.

Copper is an essential trace element that is found to be deficient in most people. It helps with oxygen and iron transportation as well as the breaking down of fat cells into energy [132]. A deficiency of copper can cause anaemia, weight gain and fertility problems [132] [195]. Copper is found in nuts, wholegrain cereals, dried prunes, avocados, artichokes, radishes, garlic, mushrooms and green vegetables. I recommend a daily dose of 1–2mg.

Dong quai (dang gui-*radix angelica sinensis*) is a herb that's used a lot in Chinese medicine to tonify the blood, regulate a woman's menstrual cycle and relieve menstrual pain [242]. It contains phytoestrogens, so should be used with caution if self-prescribing, especially by female vegetarians and vegans. Dong quai is a root and is split into three sections: the head has anticoagulant effects, the middle part is a tonic, while the tail is used to move blood stagnation. I would recommend seeing a qualified Chinese herbalist if you are considering taking this herb as it's difficult to know what part of the root is being sold in health food stores and which part would benefit your fertility.

DHA (docosahexaenoic) is an omega-3 essential fatty acid. DHA appears to be essential in brain development and growth, ultimately affecting learning abilities [240]. Around 50 per cent of the baby's brain is formed during the foetal stage, while the remaining 50 per cent is formed in the first year of birth. It is therefore important to maintain good level of DHA before conception. DHA has been shown to improve semen quality by reducing damage caused by free radicals [243]. Vegans tend to be deficient in DHA [244]. Consumption of polyunsaturated vegetable oil (omega-6) can prevent the formation of DHA. Good sources of omega-3 are oily fish, walnuts and flaxseed. I recommend a daily dose of 500mg or a daily dose of 14g (1 tablespoon) of flaxseed oil a day for vegetarians and vegans.

DHEA (dehydroepiandrosterone) is a natural hormone that exists in both men and women and increases male and female hormones. It decreases with age. Research has shown that it can improve egg quality and reduce chromosome abnormalities [31] [33] [34] [245]. The daily dose ranges from 25 to 75mg a day. Do not take DHEA in doses higher than 75–100mg a day. Eating liquorice can increase the effects of DHEA in the body [246]. Do not take if you have a family history of cancer, thyroid disorder, autism or have high testosterone levels. I would recommend speaking with your fertility doctor and testing your testosterone levels before taking this supplement. As this is a hormone, it may cause an irregular menstrual cycle and cysts which can burst mid-cycle, causing unexplained bleeding. If this should occur, stop use.

Folic acid (vitamin B$_9$) is well known for its benefits in fertility and is the only supplement recommended by Western medicine, yet only 26-28 per cent of women take it when pregnant [247] [248]. It not only helps to prevent a form of anaemia but also prevents birth defects such as spina bifida when taken during the first few weeks of pregnancy. New research has found that mothers who don't have enough folic acid in their body at the time of conception increase the risk of their baby developing autism [249], while other research has shown continued taking of folic acid into pregnancy reduces language development problems in the child [250]. Folic acid is found in green leafy vegetables and whole grains. I recommend a daily dose of 400mcg (4mg).

Ginseng *(panax ginseng)* is a root herb that boosts energy levels, similar to maca [251]. It's widely used in East Asia to boost qi levels and the digestive system, thereby helping the body produce more blood and absorb vital nutrients [242]. Research has shown that ginseng can regulate levels of leptin and normalise hypothalamus function [204] [252] [253], regulating fertility hormones. Ginseng has also been shown in research to regulate cytokines and increase levels of TH2, which protects an embryo implanting into the uterus lining [335] [336]. I recommend a daily dose of 1-3g.

Green tea. Green, white and black teas all come from the same shrub: *camellia sinensis.* Black tea is fermented green tea. The antioxidants in green tea extracts are 100 times more powerful than vitamin C and 25 times more powerful than vitamin E. It can help reduce excessive weight, blood pressure and blood stickiness, thereby improving fertility [231]. However, green tea contains caffeine which can increase levels of SHBG, which reduce free testosterone levels needed for egg and sperm development [346]. Green tea can affect the absorption of calcium. It also contains tannin, which can affect the absorption of iron. I would therefore limit drinking tea to a few cups a day and decaf if possible.

Horny goat weed is used in Chinese herbal medicine under the name of 'yin yang huo' (*herba epimedii*). Its traditional use in Chinese medicine is to improve male and female libido and fertility [242]. Research has shown that horny goat weed can restore levels of both testosterone and thyroid hormones to their normal levels [254]. I recommend a daily dose of 1000mg.

Iodine is an essential trace element that is vital for the production of two thyroid hormones thyroxin (T_4) and tri-iodothyronine (T_3) [231]. A deficiency of iodine may lead to an underactive thyroid and in newborns a condition called cretinism [231]. In conjunction with iron, it helps to replace blood loss that occurs during menstruation. Vegetarians and vegans tend to be deficient in iodine [197]. Iodine is found in fish, seaweed and unrefined sea salt. Most salts are refined and have been stripped of nearly all their 60 trace elements and replaced with fortified iodine. Try to use natural salt that hasn't been refined or altered. I recommend a daily dose of 150mcg.

Iron is an essential mineral needed for the production of haemoglobin, the red blood pigment which transports oxygen and carbon dioxide around the body. Vegetarians, vegans, menstruating and pregnant women tend to be deficient in iron [105]. Iron requirements double during pregnancy as a mother's red blood cell and haemoglobin count increases by 30 per cent. Iron, together with vitamin B_{12} and folic acid, is needed to increase blood levels. To absorb iron, there needs to be adequate levels of copper, B vitamins and vitamin C. Caffeine reduces the absorption of iron [191]. When taking iron supplements, stools may turn darker in colour, which is normal. If constipation occurs, try taking an iron supplement labelled 'gentle'. Iron is found in red meat, sardines, wheat germ, egg yolks, green vegetables and dried fruit. I recommend a daily dose of 18mg increasing to 27mg when pregnant. If your blood test comes back as iron deficient (ferritin ug/litre <30), I recommended a daily dose of 100mg.

L-arginine is an amino acid that can help improve fertility in women and sperm health in men [255]. L-arginine forms the basis of nitric oxide. Nitric oxide is found in sperm and is needed for good motility [256]. Seminal fluids contain around 25 per cent l-arginine. It also aids blood flow to the penis thereby improving erectile function [231]. Research has shown that it improves implantation and pregnancy rates [257]. L-arginine is found in nuts, seeds, pulses, beetroot, onions, grapes, rice, egg yolks and red meat. Do not take if you have PCOS or diabetes. I recommend a daily dose of 15g.

Lycopene is a powerful antioxidant, more so than beta-carotene. It has been shown to increase sperm count, motility and morphology, and reduce DNA damage [258] [259]. It is found in tomatoes, watermelon, pink grapefruit and other fruits with a red colour. It is best absorbed when heated – cooked tomatoes release five times as much as raw tomatoes. Adding olive oil increases the absorption of lycopene by three-fold [231]. I recommend a daily dose of 5-10mg [224] [258].

Maca *(lepidium meyenii)* is often referred to as 'Peruvian ginseng'. It increases energy levels and stamina and is used as an aphrodisiac [231]. Research has shown it to be of benefit to male sex drive, sexual performance, sperm count and motility, while in women it may increase luteinising hormone (LH) levels, when taken in high doses (50–100g a day) [260]. Traditional dosage of maca in the Andes of South America ranges from 50 to100g a day. I recommend a daily dose of 10g for better energy and 50g a day for those with male infertility or women with low LH levels.

Magnesium is the fourth most common mineral found in the body and yet deficiencies are common. It is needed for the function of over 300 enzymes. A deficiency of magnesium can lead to cell death. Amongst its uses is its ability to regulate the interaction of fertility hormones to their receptors [261]. Dark chocolate (70 per cent cocoa solids) contains high levels of magnesium. Magnesium is also found in beans, nuts, whole grains, seafood and dark green, leafy vegetables. I recommend a daily dose of 375mg.

Manganese is an essential mineral that has several roles, including the production of fertility hormones and blood clotting [231]. A deficiency is related to blood type deficiencies within Chinese medicine, including poor memory, nails and hair, and infertility. Manganese is found in black

(English) tea, whole grains, nuts, seeds, fruit, eggs, milk and green leafy vegetables. I recommend a daily dose of 2mg.

Melatonin is a powerful antioxidant produced by the pineal gland. It reduces levels of free radicals, which can damage egg and sperm quality [113]. It is also thought to regulate fertility hormone release from the hypothalamus [110]. Melatonin production decreases with age [113]. It is mainly produced at night when we sleep, therefore sleeping enough (7–8 hours) can help to maintain good levels. Melatonin is found in foods such as tomatoes [191]. Within the body, high concentrations are found in the female reproductive organs. Drugs such as aspirin and nonsteroidal anti-inflammatory drugs (NSAIDs) can reduce the pineal gland's production of melatonin by 75 per cent [170] [191]. I recommend a daily dose of 3mg. For women over the age of 39, on aspirin or suffering from poor sleep, I recommend a daily dose of 5mg.

Myo-inositol is a B-complex vitamin that's useful for improving egg maturation in women with poor egg quality or PCOS [262] [263] [264] [265]. Myo-inositol maybe a useful alternative in the treatment of PCOS to Metformin, which is often prescribed by doctors in the treatment of PCOS, although it's not licensed for this, has side effects, and doesn't work according to leading fertility experts [36] [266]. Myo-inositol is found in both meat and plants, but I recommend sourcing it from plants. It is found in fruits, beans, grains, and nuts. Fresh vegetables and fruits contain more myo-inositol than frozen, tinned or salt-free products. I recommend a daily dose of 250–500mg.

Nicotinamide mononucleotide (NMN) is a precursor to nicotinamide adenine dinucleotide (NAD). Levels of NAD decrease in older women. Taking NMN rejuvenates egg quality in aging females, leading to a restoration in their fertility [358]. I recommend a daily dose of 250mg and 500mg if you have poor egg quality.

Passionflower *(passiflora incarnata)* has been shown in research to improve male libido, increase sperm count and fertilisation [69]. It contains apigenin, which can increase testosterone levels. I recommend a daily dose of 100mg.

Pyrroloquinoline quinone (PQQ) s a vitamin-like substance that create more mitochondria (the energy factory of a cell). Preliminary research in animals has shown that it can improve fertility and the growth of offspring [267]. I recommend a daily dose of 20mg.

Royal jelly, also known as bee's milk, is the sole food of the queen bee and baby bees. It is a potent energy source, rich in vitamins B_5, A, C, D and E, plus amino acids, essential fatty acids, acetylcholine and minerals such as potassium, calcium, zinc, iron and manganese [231]. In Chinese medicine, it helps improve jing, yin and blood levels, while strengthening the reproductive systems in both men and women. I recommend a daily dose of 100mg.

Selenium is considered the most important trace element in our diet. It is important for both male and female fertility [224] [268]. Low levels have been linked with miscarriage and pre-eclampsia, while in men it can help with poor sperm motility [231] [243]. Selenium is found in Brazil nuts, fish, poultry, meats, whole grains, mushrooms, onions, garlic, broccoli and cabbage. Selenium is lost each time a man ejaculates. I recommend a daily dose of 200mcg.

Spirulina is a super food and known as blue-green algae (*arthrospira platensis*). It's packed full of protein with more than 60 per cent per 100g. It contains high levels of iron and vitamin B_{12}, all the essential amino acids as well as essential minerals and vitamins. It contains 180 per cent more calcium than whole milk, 670 per cent more protein than tofu, 3100 per cent more beta-carotene than carrots and 5100 per cent more iron than spinach. However, studies suggest that taking spirulina can increase TH1 cytokines, which can affect implantation of the embryo into the uterus wall [269] [270]. I would therefore recommend only men take this supplement, as it's a great substitute for meat. I recommend a daily dose of 5g in tablet form, as it doesn't taste nice in its natural powder state.

Tribulus terrestris is a plant that grows in the Mediterranean and in subtropical desert regions around the world including India and Myanmar. It's used in Ayurveda for male virility [191]. Research has shown that it can increase levels of testosterone and dihydrotestosterone which can improve semen count and motility [221]. I recommend a daily dose of 250mg.

Turmeric contains an anti-inflammatory antioxidant called curcumin that increases liver function [231]. Due to its anti-inflammatory properties, it is particularly useful in women with endometriosis [271] [272] [273] [274]. Turmeric can be combined with bromelain to improve absorption and increase the treatment of endometriosis [231]. Turmeric is yang in Nature and can help to move blood stasis, which is a common cause of endometriosis. If you have endometriosis, I recommend a daily dose of 1000mg.

Ubiquinol (ubiquinone) is the activated form of coenzyme Q10. It is a powerful antioxidant that reduces oxidative stress, thereby improving the menstrual cycle and increasing levels of follicle stimulating hormone (FSH) and LH [275]. I recommend a daily dose of 200-300mg.

Vitamin A is important in maintaining sexual health and fertility. However, it is important not to exceed the daily dose when pregnant, especially during the first seven weeks [231]. Taking more than the recommended dose can increase the risk of birth defects. Foods that contain high levels of vitamin A include fish oils (cod liver oil), liver, pâtés and fortified foods such as cereals and flour. I recommend a daily dose of 600mcg (800 RE). You can take beta-carotene instead as it can be converted into vitamin A when the body needs it, thereby reducing the chances of overdosing.

Vitamin B_1 (thiamin) is needed for the production of energy and red blood cells. The body can only store it for one month. It is present in lots of foods, however food preparation drastically decreases levels of vitamin B_1 (for example, meat that has been frozen loses 50 per cent of vitamin B_1) [231]. Vitamin B_1 can be found in whole grains, oats, meat, seafood and nuts. This vitamin is destroyed by drinking large amounts of tea or coffee. I recommend a daily dose of 1.5–2mg.

Vitamin B$_{12}$ (cobalamin) can be stored in the liver for several years, however vegetarians, and especially vegans, tend to be deficient in it [231]. In conjunction with folic acid it is needed when new genetic material is made during cell division, which helps to prevent birth defects such as spina bifida [231]. It also benefits men with a low sperm count. Vitamin B$_{12}$ can be found in oily fish, such as sardines, red meat, white fish, eggs and dairy products. I recommend a daily dose of 3–5mcg.

Vitamin B$_2$ (riboflavin) is important in the production of energy and the metabolism of proteins, fats and carbohydrates. It is needed to convert B$_6$ into its active form and helps with PMS [231]. Vitamin B$_2$ can be found in whole grains, eggs, dairy products, green leafy vegetables and beans. This is the vitamin that turns urine into a bright yellow colour [231]. I recommend a daily dose of 1.6mg.

Vitamin B$_3$ (niacin) is important in the production of energy and the use of oxygen in cells. Vitamin B$_3$ can be found in whole grains, nuts, meats, poultry, oily fish, eggs, dairy products and dried fruit. I recommend a daily dose of 15–20mg.

Vitamin B$_5$ (pantothenic acid) is important in the production of energy and adrenal gland hormones during stressful times. Vitamin B$_5$ can be found in whole grains, beans, eggs, nuts, green leafy vegetables, meats and royal jelly. I recommend a daily dose of 6mg.

Vitamin B$_6$ (pyridoxine) is essential for the action of over 60 enzymes and can help with PMS [231]. Vitamin B$_6$ can be found in whole grains, meat, oily fish, bananas, nuts, green leafy vegetables, avocados and egg yolks. I recommend a daily dose of 2mg.

Vitamin C (ascorbic acid) cannot be stored in the body so regular intake is necessary. It is needed for over 300 metabolic reactions and is vital for reproduction [231]. It helps with the absorption of iron. It is important in protecting sperm health by stopping it from clumping together and protecting the sperm's DNA [276]. Research has shown that taking vitamin C daily can increase semen quality [224]. As vitamin C is a powerful antioxidant it reduces free radical damage to eggs and sperm and benefits implantation. Vitamin C is found in most fruit and vegetables, including green leafy vegetables. I recommend a daily dose of 1g [136].

Vitamin D is found in five different forms (1, 2, 3, 4 and 5). Some vitamin D_3 is made from sunlight when the UV index is higher than three, and when not using sunscreen [231] [277]. Due to the risk of skin cancer caused by too much sun exposure, it is recommended to expose the skin to 10–15 minutes of sunlight before applying sunscreen. Most people living in cloudy countries, such as the UK, Ireland and New Zealand and the east coast of America, will have low levels of vitamin D. Even low sunscreens such as factor 8 reduce vitamin D production by 95 per cent [231] [277]. Vitamin D regulates the absorption of zinc, calcium and iron and low levels have been linked to anaemia. Vitamin D is found in sardines, herring, salmon, eggs and butter. Research has shown that women with lower levels of vitamin D have reduced fertility [192]. I recommend a daily dose of 15mcg of vitamin D_3 (cholecalciferol) in the summer months and 20mcg in the winter months.

Vitamin E is an antioxidant that protects sperm and eggs from free radical damage and is important in antibody production. Vitamin E is good for men with poor sperm motility and egg fertilisation [136]. Vitamin E can be found in wheat germ oil, eggs, spinach, leafy greens, Brussels sprouts, walnuts, pecans, avocados and butter. I recommend a daily dose of 12–15mg for females and 100-400mg for males with poor sperm motility [225].

Vitamin K is found in three different forms 1, 2 and 3. Ninety per cent of our daily intake is in the form of vitamin K1 [231]. It is essential for normal blood clotting. A deficiency can lead to heavy periods and bruising easily. Vitamin K can be found in cauliflower, broccoli, dark green, leafy vegetables, egg yolks, safflower, kelp, yoghurt, rapeseed, olive oils, tomatoes, red meat and potatoes. I recommend a daily dose of 100mcg.

Zinc is an important mineral for male and female fertility as it plays a crucial role in the sensitivity of bodily tissues to circulating fertility hormones. It is vital for sexual maturity. Zinc deficiencies in females can lead to irregular levels of FSH and LH [278]. A deficiency of zinc can lead to low testosterone levels and delayed male puberty [279]. Each ejaculation of semen contains around 110mg of zinc, therefore excessive sperm loss or a poor diet can lead to a deficiency of zinc. Zinc is important in sperm health as it helps to maintain the DNA in the sperm head, while also ensuring the sperm do not become too excited and release the enzyme acrosome (which breaks down the egg wall, helping the sperm enter and fertilise the egg) before a woman's egg is released [280]. During fertilisation, zinc is released which causes a 'zinc spark': a flash of light at the moment of conception [281]. Zinc can be found in red meat, pumpkin seeds, whole grains, ground mustard, eggs and cheese. I recommend a daily dose of 15mg for men and women. Men with a low sperm count can take up to 66mg [137].

Part Five

Aiding Natural Conception

The use of alternative therapies in fertility treatment is growing rapidly as people try to find solutions and ways around their fertility problems. There is a growing body of research that supports the use of acupuncture in the treatment of male and female infertility (see page 206).

How long should I try for naturally?

The length of time you want to try naturally is a personal choice but should be viewed in a critical manner. Knowing when you are at your physical, mental and emotional best and have optimised your lifestyle and diet – and tried naturally long enough – is important in knowing when to move on to another route. A lot of people tend to try IVF without getting their body ready for natural conception to occur first.

If you feel that you have tried long enough, for example for more than one year after following the recommendations within this book, then you may decide to try another route, for example assisted reproduction techniques such as Clomid (see Chapter Fifteen). Before jumping to Clomid, make sure you have tried acupuncture and Chinese herbal medicine for at least three to four months first [125].

Chapter 13

Acupuncture All the Way!

Acupuncture is one of the most popular alternative therapies for infertility. Acupuncture does more than just relax people; it balances the hypothalamus, thereby enhancing fertility hormones from the pituitary gland as well as regulating energy and blood flow within the body, which helps to normalise fertility hormones contained within the blood. All this helps to regulate the menstrual cycle. It is the menstrual cycle that is the most important aspect of fertility treatment within Chinese medicine. Since around 95 per cent of women experience premenstrual symptoms [282], such as sweating at night, abdominal cramps, pain, tender breasts, lower back pain and premenstrual syndrome (PMS/PMT), they are considered normal, but they are not. In Chinese medicine these are all abnormal and give insights into what internal imbalance a woman might have.

Research has shown that having acupuncture weekly for nine weeks reduced the time to conception by half [283]. It helps to better your health and improve your fertility and that of your baby, as their fertility is determined in part by your health at the time of conception. This is important because second generation women born from mothers who had fertility treatment are showing inherited premature infertility (IPI), a syndrome whereby their fertility is reduced by several years, leaving them struggling to have a child at a younger age than their mothers. This can have a knock-on effect on future generations.

History of acupuncture

Acupuncture is often viewed as a strange form of therapy originating from East Asia where they are all Buddhists. This is far from the truth! There is now some proof with the discovery of the frozen Oetzi tattoo man found in the Italian Alps in 1991 that acupuncture may have been around in Europe over 5000 years ago [284]. Therefore acupuncture doesn't necessarily belong to East Asia. What is known is that its use has been well-documented in East Asia for over 2000 years and has a long and successful history. When people think of acupuncture, they tend to think of China. However, acupuncture has been practised all over East Asia, including Japan, Korea and Vietnam. It is therefore not the sole property of the Chinese, though they had the most influence in its development.

Acupuncture probably originated in ancient times through massage (acupressure and scraping), when people would massage a point on the body and found that it helped another part of the body that was in discomfort. People in East Asia then added their unique understanding and awareness of Nature to these points to give us the acupuncture we know today.

The technology used to make acupuncture needles, or rather pins, has evolved over the centuries from stone, to thick needles to the ultra-fine pins we use today [285]. They are as fine as a human hair and you can fit 20 acupuncture pins into just one syringe. In the West, these ultra-fine pins are just used once and then put into a special container (sharps box) that is incinerated for health and safety reasons.

A country's success is greatly influenced by the medicine it uses. Its birth rate, child death rate, general health level and how long the population lives for are all largely dependent upon the healthcare system practised within that country. The Chinese population are successful in all these areas of life, due to their cultural awareness of Nature, diet, lifestyle and the medicine they use. It's therefore no wonder the Chinese have the largest population in the world and have had to implement birth control measures to keep population numbers down. This is largely thanks to Chinese medicine.

Is acupuncture safe?

A large-scale study published in 2009 found acupuncture to be very safe after reviewing over 229,230 treatments [286]. However, in most Western countries, doctors, physiotherapists, osteopaths, chiropractors, nurses and massage therapists can legally perform 'acupuncture' after just a short course. It's not possible to learn over 2000 years of medicine in a few weekends. This can have an effect upon the safety and effectiveness of the acupuncture treatment. Therefore, I would recommend only having acupuncture from a properly trained acupuncturist.

How does acupuncture work?

Acupuncture is made up of points on the body where the energy can be influenced. These points connect together to form the channels (meridians). These channels look like the underground (tube or metro) map, with lots of different lines crisscrossing each other. The stations are like the acupuncture points. Each point has an associated health property. By inserting a pin into the acupuncture point, it tells the body to initiate a healing response.

Acupuncture is good at helping to regulate energy and blood flow throughout the body. When these two important aspects of the body are regulated, the body is able to heal itself and return to a state of balance, known as 'homeostasis' in Western medicine. During an acupuncture session, the patient will often go into a deep state of relaxation where they are able to switch off from their worries and stresses, allowing the body to heal itself.

Today there are currently two theories as to how acupuncture works and what makes up the acupuncture points and channels. Within Western medical thinking, it is believed acupuncture works on the nervous system, hence its ability to relieve pain. However, this theory isn't recognised within the acupuncture community, or in East Asia, because acupuncture is able to do a lot more than just relieve pain. A better theory originates from Korea, where researchers believe they have found the channels anatomically within the body [287]. They believe they have observed the actual channels running within the lymphatic (immune) system [115]. Other research conducted in Belgium also found the same structures [288]. Additional research into the pathways of free radicals (reactive oxygen species) found that the chain reaction of free radicals moved long the same pathways of the immune system as the acupuncture channels [114].

Does it hurt?

Some people don't like the idea of needles and worry that acupuncture will hurt. This fear of needles normally comes from bad memories after having a blood test or a vaccination. Having acupuncture isn't the same as having a blood test, as the acupuncture pin is a lot thinner and isn't inserted into a vein but rather a muscle.

Some people will feel the acupuncture pins more than others. This is often due to a lack of energy. The weaker the person is, the more sensitive they are and the more they will feel the pin breaking the skin, causing a quick prick sensation. When the pin hits the acupuncture point, the sensations a person can feel are unlike anything you've normally felt and can be:

- a dull throbbing ache
- a pulling sensation
- a tingling sensation
- an electrical sensation that travels along the body

Research-proven benefits of acupuncture for fertility

Unlike most alternative therapies, there has been a lot of new research into the use of acupuncture that has confirmed its beneficial effects upon male and female fertility. Acupuncture has been shown in research studies to:

- enhance the effects of clomiphene citrate [62]
- improve implantation by increasing the uterus receptibility [62] [289] [357]
- improve ovarian reserve [290]
- improve sensitivity to insulin [291]
- improve sperm motility, morphology and quality [292] [293] [294] [295] [296] [297]
- increase antral follicle count [51]
- increase blood flow to the uterus [7] [298] [299] [300]
- reduce anxiety, stress and depression [6] [301] [302]
- reduce insomnia and increase melatonin levels [337]
- reduce high follicle stimulating hormone (FSH) levels [27] [290]
- reduce uterine contractions [303] [304]
- reduce weight [131]
- regulate AMH levels [27]
- regulate immune factors, i.e. TH1/TH2, NK cells and cytokines [64] [305] [306] [307] [308] [309]
- regulate luteinising hormone (LH) levels [310]
- regulate oestrogen levels [62] [311]
- regulate the menstrual cycle [7] [8] [44]
- regulate the stress hormone cortisol [146]
- stimulate ovulation [8] [312]

What will I feel after having acupuncture?

The most noticeable effect people feel after having acupuncture treatment is how calm and relaxed they are. However, that's not all. Some people say they feel a bit light-headed after getting off the couch, which is normal. Some even sleep during acupuncture treatment, which can give the person a great catnap and restore their energy levels. I find that the more the person relaxes on the couch, the better the acupuncture works. After having acupuncture, it is generally safe to drive or go back to work or exercise. Most people like to have acupuncture after work as they often feel too relaxed to want to go back to their desk again!

When should I have acupuncture in my cycle?

It is beneficial to have acupuncture during most parts of your menstrual cycle. Personally, I don't believe it's necessary to have acupuncture when you're bleeding heavily at the start of your menstrual cycle because your FSH levels are still low and you may be more sensitive to the pins being inserted. From around day 4–5 of your cycle, when FSH levels start to rise, having acupuncture can help with follicle growth and maturation. Once ovulation has occurred, acupuncture can help with implantation 5–7 days afterwards. During the last week of the menstrual cycle, acupuncture can help with the anxiety and emotional stress of wondering whether you are pregnant.

How often do I need to have acupuncture?

Acupuncture is a dose like every other medical treatment. Its effects last for around 3–4 days and then it needs to be repeated. It is ideal to have acupuncture twice a week. Due to financial constraints, some people will opt to have acupuncture once a week. Having acupuncture less frequently than once a week is not advisable because its effects will be minimal.

How long should I have acupuncture for?

If you fall pregnant naturally, you should continue having acupuncture until at least 12 weeks. However, some women like to have acupuncture for longer to help with anxiety and ensure the pregnancy carries on smoothly, which is good for the mother and the baby as any problems can be picked up before they develop further. Having acupuncture throughout the whole pregnancy is ideal.

If you have a low anti-Müllerian hormone (AMH) level or are over the age of 40, I would recommend having acupuncture throughout the whole pregnancy. You will often be weaker and the pregnancy more precious, so every effort needs to be utilised to maintain the pregnancy.

Chapter 14

Chinese Herbs

Chinese herbs are often overlooked in fertility treatment. This is because most people are unaware of their benefits. Also most acupuncturists can't offer herbs as they don't practise herbal medicine (which is alien to the Chinese). The use of herbs in fertility treatment can greatly benefit both male and female fertility. This can sometimes be the deciding factor as to whether a couple ends up having a baby. I know I am biased, but I recommend herbs to most of my patients. I take them daily myself, as does my partner who was pregnant when I first started writing this book.

History of Chinese herbs

Herbs have been used to treat various health problems all over the world, including Europe, the Americas, Africa and Asia, for tens of thousands of years. In the West, the word 'medicine' used to mean herbal medicine. It's only in the last 125 years, since aspirin was extracted from the bark of the willow tree [313], that pharmaceutical drugs have become more and more popular and the use of plants has become less so.

Pharmaceutical drugs are often the synthesised active ingredients of plants. A quarter of all pharmaceutical drugs originate from plants [314].

The active ingredient is then patented and its potency increased many times over to make it very effective and quick-working. However, as it's just one part of the original plant, it's no longer part of Nature and as *we* are still part of Nature, it causes us side effects. If the original herbs are used instead, the actions take longer to work but seldom have side effects. Herbal medicine is really the traditional medicine of the world and the use of pharmacological drugs is a newer alternative.

How can herbs help fertility?

It's not often known that in China people opt for herbs first before trying acupuncture. This is because herbs are more powerful and can fix a fertility problem a lot quicker. In the West, it's the opposite, as acupuncture gets more press so tends to be more popular than herbs. In terms of fertility, it's best to have both, so try to find a practitioner that practises both acupuncture and Chinese herbal medicine.

Research conducted in 2011 found that the management of female infertility with Chinese herbal medicine can improve pregnancy rates two-fold within a four-month period compared with Western medical fertility drug therapy or IVF [125]. They found that assessment of the quality of the menstrual cycle, integral to traditional Chinese medicine diagnosis, appeared to be fundamental to the successful treatment of female infertility. Other research has shown that Chinese herbal formulas, such as Bu Shen Tiao Chong Tang, have the same effect on ovaries as IVF drugs [315]. Another Chinese herbal formula – Bu Shen Sheng Jiang Pian – has been shown to regulate levels of follicle stimulating hormone (FSH), prolactin, testosterone and corticosterone, thereby improving male fertility [316], while another Chinese herbal formula – Bu Zhong Yi Qi Tang – has been shown in research conducted in Japan to reduce sperm motility issues by over 50 per cent [317]. Chinese herbs can also help with male infertility caused by circulation disorders in varicocele (an enlargement of the veins within the loose bag of skin that holds the testicles) [318] [319]. Another

Chinese herbal formula – Wen Jing Tang – has been found to regulate levels of luteinising hormone (LH) [320], while Xiao Yao Wan can improve pregnancy rates in women with tubal infertility [321]. Individual herbs have also been tested in research studies, for example Shan Zhu Yu (*cornus officinalis*) was found to increase sperm motility [322].

Is it safe to take herbs?

When herbs are prescribed by a qualified herbalist, they are largely safe – often safer than pharmaceutical drugs. However, Chinese herbs tend to get a lot of bad press. We often hear negative stories such as endangered species or steroids being found in Chinese herbs. As medicine in China was unified in the 1950s [323], both Western pharmaceuticals and Chinese herbs are used together, so a single pill will contain both types of medicine (pharmaceutical agents and herbs) to make it a lot more effective. Unfortunately, some of these pills were shipped to Western countries, where the medicine is not unified, causing problems and bad press.

The use of Chinese herbs in Western countries is now tightly controlled and all the herbs imported are monitored for quality. In rare news stories, we hear of people suffering from kidney failure or even death after taking herbs. These types of stories make headline news, while the 237 million medical mistakes made a year in the UK don't [324]. Around 62,000 people are admitted to hospital every year in the UK from adverse reactions to pharmaceutical drugs [325] and medical errors are the third biggest killer of people in the USA [326].

Side effects from herbs are not common. Deaths from taking herbs are very rare. However, the wrong herbs in the wrong hands (those that aren't taught or licensed to prepare herbs) can potentially cause problems. Always see a properly qualified herbalist.

What will I feel after taking herbs?

When people visit my clinic for fertility treatment, they usually talk about other problems they might have, for example feeling cold or dizzy, or having poor sleep or a sluggish digestion. After discussing their case, they often realise that all their problems are connected and related to each other, and then it all makes sense. Once people start taking herbs, they often notice that their other symptoms, such as being cold, dizzy or tired, have gone, making them feel better. This is because Chinese medicine sees the person as a whole and not as different segments that different specialist doctors need to treat. This departmentalisation in Western medicine often means that one department is unaware of the other department and how related they are to each other, sadly to the detriment of the patient's health.

How do you take herbs?

Traditionally herbs come in their raw form, for example bits of root, bark, seeds or flower heads that you would cook in water then drain and drink. This process takes hours, can stink your kitchen out and leaves sediment at the bottom of your cup, which can make you gag when you drink it. Nowadays, it's a lot easier. The herbs come in powder form so you don't need to spend hours cooking them. Instead you just add hot water and honey, wait for them to cool down and then drink. They often don't taste nice, hence the honey. Some of my patients prefer to have them in tablet form, which have no bad taste at all. Herbs are generally taken twice a day, in the morning and evening, allowing the beneficial actions of the herbs to be spread out throughout the day.

Dosages

There are two dosages in Chinese herbal medicine: the raw herbs/powders and small black pills. The small black pills are standard off-the-shelf formulas at a very weak dose. You can buy them online or in health food stores; however, they are illegal in Europe. I don't recommend using them as they are too weak, take a long time to work and cannot be customised to a person's individual needs. A lot of people are attracted to them because they are cheap. I don't recommend self-diagnosing or self-treating using Chinese herbs. Prescribing an accurate and effective formula is an art form that takes many years of study and practise. If you want to take Chinese herbs, only buy them from a well-qualified herbalist after having a consultation.

How long do I need to take herbs?

You can take Chinese herbs before falling pregnant and throughout pregnancy. They are perfectly safe to take and will help the foetus grow and ensure you have good levels of energy and blood needed for breastfeeding. Taking Chinese herbs will also reduce any side effects the pregnancy may have upon your body, for example depression (baby blues), anxiety and physical depletion.

Chapter 15

Assisted Natural Conception

If you've been on your fertility journey for a long time and are losing patience, you can use pharmaceutical drugs to help induce conception. These drugs are powerful and can be effective, but they also carry with them side effects for both the mother and baby. This is because when you force your body to do something when it isn't naturally ready, it will produce a less healthy embryo. Being aware of this will help you make a properly informed decision as to whether you want to use these medications or not.

Clomid (clomifene or clomiphene)

Clomid was developed in the 1950s and is commonly prescribed by doctors to induce ovulation. It's taken at the start of the menstrual cycle from around day 2 at a dose of 50mg daily for five days [266]. If a second course is prescribed the dose can be increased to 100mg. A course of three cycles is considered a course of treatment. It is licensed for six months' use. It is not recommended to take Clomid for more than six months [266].

Clomid works by blocking oestradiol feedback to the pituitary gland, which would normally stop follicle stimulating hormone (FSH) production, so the pituitary gland carries on releasing FSH to greatly stimulate the ovaries to produce follicles. This mechanism can bypass leptin levels which, in normal circumstances, would give the 'green light' to the hypothalamus to make the pituitary gland increase FSH production. It forces the body to produce follicles when naturally the body wouldn't as it's not strong enough, hence the side effects associated with the use of Clomid.

In Chinese medicine, Clomid is hot in nature which enhances blood flow to the follicles. It's suitable for women who feel cold (a deficiency of yang) but who don't sweat at night. If the woman feels warm or hardly ever feels the cold and can sometimes sweat at night, then Clomid is too warm and will damage yin; like being on a slow cook, it will burn and damage the body's fluids, leading to, for example, less cervical mucous. This can actually worsen a woman's fertility. It has also been shown to reduce gland development in the uterus wall, thereby damaging implantation [327]. To offset this side effect, acupuncture can be used, which research has shown stimulates the thickening of the uterus wall (uterine glandular development) thereby improving implantation [62] and improving the egg quality [328].

The side effects of Clomid in mother or baby include:

- abdominal distension
- an abnormally growth of tissue in the body (neoplasms)
- anxiety
- birth defects
- blood clot in the brain (cerebral thrombosis)
- breast tenderness
- cataract
- decreased bile flow (cholestatic)
- depression
- disorientation
- dizziness and vertigo
- fatigue
- hair loss
- headaches
- high levels of triglycerides (hypertriglyceridemia)

- hot flushes
- inflammation of the optic nerve in the eye which causes pain and poor vision (optic neuritis)
- insomnia
- jaundice
- menstrual cycle irregularities
- mood swings
- nausea and vomiting
- nervous system disorders
- ovarian and fallopian tube disorders
- palpitations
- pancreatitis
- prevent breast milk development
- psychosis
- rapid heart rate (tachycardia)
- seizures
- skin reactions
- speech disorder
- stroke
- swelling of the lower layer of skin and tissue (angioedema)
- temporary loss of consciousness caused by insufficient blood flow to the brain (syncope)
- tingling, pricking, chilling, burning, or numb sensation on the skin (paraesthesia)
- uterine disorders
- vertigo
- vision disorders [266] [329]

If you intend to go down this route and use Clomid, I would still recommend prepping yourself with the information contained within this book for three to four months first. This should help increase the success rates of Clomid and possibly reduce some of the side effects.

Intra-uterine insemination (IUI)

IUI is the injection of sperm into the woman's uterus via the cervix. It is generally painless and can be performed as an outpatient. IUI is sometimes combined with small doses of ovulation-inducing drugs, such as Clomid, to increase the success rates. In my experience, women over 40 should not try IUI as it's unlikely to succeed and is essentially wasting valuable time and money.

In a study that measured the effectiveness of both acupuncture and Chinese herbs in combination with IUI infertility treatment, the results showed a significant increase in fertility when both acupuncture and Chinese herbs were given together. Out of the 29 women in the acupuncture and Chinese herb group, 41.4 per cent delivered healthy babies. In the control group, only 26.9 per cent delivered. The vast difference in success rates is even more surprising when the age of the average woman was taken into account. The average age of the women in the acupuncture and Chinese herb group was 39.4, while that of the control group was 37.1 [330]. Normally, the older the mother, the lower the pregnancy and live birth rates.

Conclusion

I hope you have found the information within this book useful. The information is based upon the ancient theories of Chinese medicine, together with modern scientific research studies and my clinical experience treating thousands of couples with infertility.

By making lots of little changes to your diet and lifestyle, as outlined in this book, and with the added awareness of how your body works, you can take back control of your fertility and increase the chances of becoming pregnant, having your baby and being a parent.

The more information you can take from this book and utilise in your daily life, the better your chances are of having a baby. Of course, it takes two to tango, so it's important that your partner also takes on this advice and makes positive changes to their diet and lifestyle.

Even though you were born to be a parent and have millions of years of evolution behind you, some people just need a little help; a few changes here and a few changes there can be all that are needed to allow your body to rebalance itself, for everything to fall into synch allowing natural fertility to take place.

Remember, you are not alone in struggling to have your baby! More and more couples are in the same situation and there is lots of support available to you if you need it. You can use the online forum I set up for couples struggling with their fertility to gain support: visit **www.myfertilityforum.com.**

I offer couples personalised fertility plans based upon their unique infertility and health needs. I can support and offer dietary, lifestyle advice to maximise your fertility and chances of getting pregnant. In addition, I can advise on what to do next and the various options available to you. Once pregnant, I offer treatment plans to minimise problems and ensure a healthy pregnancy and labour. My treatments are available either in person at one of my private clinics or online via video.

For further information on my services, please visit **www.attiliodalberto.com.**

Fertility checklist ☑️

- ☐ Avoid plastics, chemicals and some medications.
- ☐ Be aware of the causes of infertility and how they can affect your fertility.
- ☐ Drink 2 litres (½ gallon) of water a day.
- ☐ Drink no more than two glasses of red wine (125ml/1.4 units per glass) a week.
- ☐ Eat foods that are fresh and organic.
- ☐ Eat meals from my male and female diet plans.
- ☐ Exercise (cardio) three times a week.
- ☐ Get tested to assess your fertility. Self-testing can also help you become more aware of yourself and your fertility.
- ☐ Have regular counselling to deal with trapped emotions.
- ☐ Join **www.myfertilityforum.com** to gain support.
- ☐ Listen to your body to know where you are in your menstrual cycle. Know the signs and symptoms of ovulation that are specific to you. This is important in determining when to have sex.
- ☐ Minimise your exposure to gadgets, social media and negative news stories.
- ☐ Practise yoga, mindfulness or meditation.
- ☐ Remember to have fun and enjoy what you already have.
- ☐ Seek out a fertility acupuncturist specialist who also practises herbal medicine.
- ☐ Sleep early (before 10 p.m.) and don't work night shifts.
- ☐ Take various supplements, as outlined in Chapter Twelve.
- ☐ Understand your hormones and the components of fertility.
- ☐ Wear clothes to aid blood flow.

Fertility Dictionary

Acrosome: an enzyme found in the head of a sperm that's used to break down the outer wall of an egg allowing a sperm to enter the egg.

Acupoints: specific points on the body where acupuncture pins or moxa are applied to elicit a healing response.

Acupuncture: the insertion of fine pins into acupuncture points along the channels of the body to promote good health and fertility.

Adenomyosis: a condition where the inner lining of the uterus breaks through the muscle wall of the uterus.

Adrenocorticotrophic hormone (ACTH): a hormone produced by the pituitary gland that influences the production of hormones by the adrenals.

Advanced glycation end products (AGEs): originating from sugar, AGEs affect implantation by making the uterus lining hostile.

Amenorrhoea: the absence of a menstrual period.

Androgens: are made up of testosterone, androstenedione and SHBG.

Anovulation: the absence of ovulation.

Anti-Müllerian hormone (AMH): a measure of egg reserve.

Antioxidants: a molecule that stops a chain reaction causing the creation of free radicals.

Antral follicle count (AFC): a measure of preceding follicles (potential eggs).

Asherman's syndrome: uterine scarring that prevents the regrowth of the uterus lining.

Asthenospermia (asthenozoospermia): reduced sperm motility.

Azoospermia: no sperm in the male semen.

Basal body temperature (BBT): the measuring of your body temperature at the same time every morning to determine ovulation.

Blastocyst: a 5–6-day-old fertilised embryo. A blastocyst is different from a morula as it has formed into a hollow ball with an inner cavity.

Blood stasis: the impairment of normal blood flow.

Blood: the same in both Western and Chinese medicines.

Body mass index (BMI): a mathematical equation (divide your weight in kilograms by your height in metres squared) that tries to measure a person's body fat.

Chinese herbs: different types of plants mixed together to form a therapeutic decoction to heal the person.

Chinese medicine: a system of medicine that uses observations in Nature to maintain good health. It incorporates acupuncture, herbal medicine, moxibustion, cupping, gua sha and tui na to rectify health problems.

Chlamydia: a sexually transmitted disease that can cause infections in the pelvis (pelvic inflammatory disease), which may affect the fallopian tubes causing ectopic pregnancies, chronic pain and infertility.

Chocolate cysts: blood-filled cysts.

Clomid: also known as clomifene citrate, is a drug used to try to induce ovulation.

CMV: cytomegalovirus, a herpes virus, which can cause birth defects.

Corpus luteum: the formation of the collapsed follicle (egg) sac, which releases progesterone.

Corticotrophic-releasing hormone (CRH): affects levels of the stress hormone cortisone.

Cretinism: mental and physical retardation due to hypothyroidism brought about by a lack of iodine in the pregnant mother.

Cyst: a sac-like pocket of tissue that contains fluid, air or other substances.

Cytokines: proteins produced by the immune system that affect the behaviour of immune cells, which can affect implantation and the development of the fertilised embryo.

D&C: dilatation and curettage to remove an embryo from the uterus.

Dampness: similar to fog and the wet nature of woods and forests.

Dehydroepiandrosterone (DHEA): a naturally occurring steroid that can enhance egg quality.

Dermoid cyst: a small collection of bodily tissues, such as hair, teeth, blood, bone, fat, eyes, etc.

Dysmenorrhoea: pain during the menstrual bleed.

E2: oestradiol.

ELISA: 'enzyme linked immunosorbent assay', which is used to test for antibodies in relation to certain infections, i.e. hepatitis C.

Embryo: a fertilised egg.

Endometriosis: when the lining of the uterus starts to grow in other places, such as the ovaries and fallopian tubes.

Endometrium/endometrial: the lining of the uterus (womb) wall.

Endomyometritis: an infection of the uterus.

Excessive cold: the same as being too cold in Nature, such as during winter, when things move slower.

Excessive heat: the same as being too hot in Nature, such as in the height of summer when it's too hot and we feel uncomfortable, restless and thirsty.

Fallopian tubes: the tubes that join the ovaries to the uterus.

Fibroids: non-cancerous tumours, made up of muscle and fibrous tissue that grow in or around the uterus in various sizes.

Five elements: the five phases of material change: fire, earth, metal, water and wood.

Follicle stimulating hormone (FSH): released by the pituitary gland that stimulates the ovaries to produce follicles (eggs).

Follicle: the sac in which an egg grows before ovulation occurs.

Free radicals: an uncharged molecule in a cell.

Gametes: the male and female reproductive cells: sperm and egg.

Gonadotrophin-releasing hormone (GnRH): released by the hypothalamus, which causes the release of FSH and LH from the pituitary gland.

Gonorrhoea: a sexually transmitted disease that can cause infections in the pelvis (pelvic inflammatory disease), which may affect the fallopian tubes causing ectopic pregnancies, chronic pain and infertility.

Hatching: enzymes released by the blastocyst erode a hole in the uterus wall to aid implantation.

HPT: home pregnancy test.

Human chorionic gonadotrophin (hCG): released by the embedded embryo, which is used by pregnancy tests to detect pregnancy.

Hyfosy: an internal ultrasound scan using a contrast solution of sterile water and sterile inert gel.

Hyperprolactinaemia: higher than normal levels of prolactin.

Hypothalamus: the area in the brain that releases GnRH.

Hysterosalpingography: an X-ray examination of a woman's uterus and fallopian tubes that uses a special form of X-ray called fluoroscopy with a contrast material.

Hysteroscopy: the examination of the uterus using a small telescope.

Immune testing: the testing of cytokines and NK cells to determine if a woman has a hyperactive immune response, which can prevent an embryo implanting into the uterus wall.

Infertility: the inability to conceive after 12 months of regular unprotected sexual intercourse.

Inhibin: the hormone released by a mature egg that stops the release of FSH.

IPI: inherited premature infertility.

Jing: also known as 'essence'; a more concentrated form of yin that is housed in the kidneys. In men it is his semen and in women her eggs.

Laparoscopy: the examination of the pelvis using a small telescope.

Laparotomy: a large incision made through the abdominal wall to gain access into the abdominal cavity.

Leukaemia inhibitory factor (LIF): essential for implantation and produced by IL-4 cytokine. Acupuncture increases its levels.

Leydig cells: found in male testis and produce testosterone.

Lipids: organic compounds made up of fats and oils.

Liver qi stagnation: the stagnation of energy in the liver organ.

Luteinised unruptured follicle syndrome: when the egg is not released by the follicle sac following a surge of LH.

Luteinising hormone (LH): released by the pituitary gland and triggers ovulation.

Menorrhagia: a heavy bleed at the start of the menstrual cycle.

Mittelschmerz: ovulation pain with bleeding.

Morula: a 3–4-day-old fertilised embryo with an identical number of cells.

Moxa: also called moxibustion, is the use of heat therapy on specific acupoints.

Nanogram (ng): a unit of substance equal to one billionth of a gram.

NK cells: natural killer cells that form part of the immune system.

Oedema: fluid retention in areas of the body.

Oestradiol: the most abundant and dominant hormone from the group of oestrogens.

Oestrogens: the group of hormones secreted by the developing follicle.

Oligomenorrhoea: a very irregular menstrual cycle that occurs every 35 days to six months.

Oligospermia (oligozoospermia): reduced sperm concentration.

Oocyte: an egg that hasn't been fertilised.

Ovaries: the female reproductive organs containing follicles.

Ovulation: the release of the egg from the follicle sac.

P4: progesterone.

Phytoestrogens: naturally-occurring oestrogens found in plants.

Picomole (pmol): a unit of substance equal to one trillionth (10^{-12}) of a mole.

Pituitary gland: the gland that secretes FSH, LH, prolactin and oxytocin.

Placenta: an organ that connects the developing foetus to the wall of the uterus.

Polycystic ovaries (PCO): multiple cysts on the ovary without higher levels of testosterone or LH as seen in PCOS.

Polycystic ovary syndrome (PCOS): multiple cysts on the ovary with higher than normal levels of LH and testosterone.

Premenstrual syndrome (PMS): a condition when a woman feels tension, irritability, aggression, depression and a loss of control before her menstrual cycle starts. Also known as premenstrual tension (PMT).

Progesterone: the steroid hormone released by the corpus luteum, which maintains the uterus lining.

Progestins: a group of steroid hormones produced by the corpus luteum. The main progestin is progesterone.

Prolactin: stimulates breast development and lactation.

Qi: energy. Qi comes from food, sleep, tonics and qi gong.

Reactive oxygen species (ROS): a by-product of oxygen metabolism.

Sex hormone-binding globulin (SHBG): a carrier protein that binds to testosterone making it inactive.

Sperm: the male gamete.

Teratospermia (teratozoospermia): reduced sperm morphology.

Testosterone: the main male androgen hormone.

TH1: inhibit pregnancy when levels are greater than TH2.

TH2: protect pregnancy when levels are greater than TH1.

Total antioxidant capacity (TAC): used to measure the level of oxidative stress in semen.

Toxoplasmosis: a parasite that can cause infertility.

TRH: thyrotrophin-releasing hormone.

TSH: thyroid stimulating hormone.

Tubal occlusion: blocked fallopian tubes.

Tubal patency: open fallopian tubes.

Uterine lining: the lining of the uterus (womb).

Varicoceles: enlarged varicose veins that occur in areas such as the male scrotum, which can cause male infertility.

Waist–hip ratio: a more accurate measure of body fat than BMI: divide your waist measurement by your hip measurement.

Yang: a type of energy that relates to male, the sun, active, midday, hot, summer, sperm, etc.

Yin: a type of energy that relates to female, the moon, passive, midnight, cold, winter, egg, etc.

Zika virus: causes congenital birth defects.

Zona pellucida: the outer layer of an embryo.

Zygote: a newly fertilised egg.

References

1. *Obesity associated advanced glycation end products within the human uterine cavity adversely impact endometrial function and embryo implantation competence.* **Antoniotti, Gabriella , et al.,** s.l. : Human Reproduction, 2018.

2. *Psychological evaluation and support in a program of in vitro fertilization and embryo transfer.* **Freeman, EW, et al.,** 1, s.l. : Fertility and Sterility, 1985, Fertility & Sterility, Vol. 43, pp. 48-53.

3. *In vitro fertilization and breast cancer: is there cause for concern?* **Stewart, Louise, et al.,** 2, s.l. : Fertility and Sterility, 2012, Vol. 98.

4. **Magowan, Brian, Owen, Philip and Thomson, Andrew.** *Clinic Obstretics & Gynaecology.* Edinburgh : Elsevier, 2014.

5. *Relationship between hair and salivary cortisol and pregnancy in women undergoing IVF.* **Massey, Adam, et al.,** s.l. : Psychoneuroendocrinology, 2016, Vol. 74.

6. *Influence of Acupuncture on HPA Axis in a Rat Model of Chronic Stress-induced Depression.* **Sun, Dong-wei, Wang, Long and Sun, Zhong-ren.** 4, s.l. : Journal of Acupuncture and Tuina Science, 2007, Vol. 5.

7. *Role of acupuncture in the treatment of female infertility.* **Chang, Raymond, Chung, Pak and Rosenwaks, Zev .** 6, s.l. : Fertility and Sterility, 2002, Vol. 78.

8. *Acupuncture normalizes dysfunction of hypothalamic-pituitary-ovarian axis.*
    Chen, Bo-Ying. 2, s.l. : Acupuncture & Electro-Therapeutics Research, 1997,
    Vol. 22.

9. *Age-specific FSH levels as a tool for appropriate patient counselling in assisted
    reproduction.* **Weghofer, Andrea , et al.,** 9, s.l. : Human Reproduction, 2005,
    Vol. 20.

10. *Age-Specific Levels for Basal Follicle Stimulating Hormone Assessment of Ovarian
    Function.* **Barad, David, Weghofer, Andrea and Gleicher, Norbert.** 6, s.l. :
    Obstetrics & Gynecology, 2007, Vol. 109.

11. *Gestational stress, placental norepinephrine transporter and offspring fertility.*
    Piquer, Beatriz , Fonseca, Jose and Lara , Hernán. 2, s.l. : Reproduction,
    2017, Vol. 153.

12. *Rotating Shift Work and Menstrual Cycle Characteristics.* **Lawson, Christina, et
    al.,** 2011, Epidemiology, pp. 305-312.

13. **Beckmann, Charles, et al.,** *Obstretics and Gynecology.* Philadelphia : Wolters
    Kluwer, 2010.

14. *Evidence for GnRH Regulation by Leptin: Leptin Administration Prevents
    Reduced Pulsatile LH Secretion during Fasting.* **Nagatan, Shoji, et al.,** s.l. :
    Neuroendocrinology, 1998, Vol. 67.

15. *Microbial Reconstitution Reverses Maternal Diet-Induced Social and Synaptic
    Deficits in Offspring.* **Buffington, S A, et al.,** 7, s.l. : Cell, 2016, Vol. 165.

16. *The Fat-Induced Satiety Factor Oleoylethanolamide Suppresses Feeding through
    Central Release of Oxytocin.* **Gaetani, Silvana, et al.,** 24, s.l. : The Journal of
    Neuroscience, 2010, Vol. 30.

17. *Peripheral oxytocin treatment ameliorates obesity by reducing food intake and
    visceral fat mass.* **Maejima, Yuko and Iwasaki, Yusaku .** 12, s.l. : Aging, 2011,
    Vol. 3.

18. *The antinociceptive effect of non-noxious sensory stimulation is mediated partly
    through oxytocinergic mechanisms.* **Uvnäs-Moberg, K, et al.,** 2, s.l. : Acta
    Physiol Scand, 1993, Vol. 149.

19. *Stress and outcome success in IVF: the role of self-reports and endocrine variables.* **Smeenk, J, et al.,** 4, s.l. : Human Reproduction, 2005, Vol. 20.

20. *Ferrous Sulfate Reduces Thyroxine Efficacy in Patients with Hypothyroidism.* **Campbell, Norman, et al.,** 12, s.l. : Ann Intern Med, 1992, Vol. 117.

21. *Effect of Calcium Carbonate on the Absorption of Levothyroxine.* **Singh, Nalini , Singh, Pramil and Hershman, Jerome.** 21, s.l. : JAMA, 2000, Vol. 283.

22. *Testing and interpreting measures of ovarian reserve: a committee opinion.* **Practice Committee of the American Society for Reproductive Medicine.** 3, s.l. : Fertility and Sterility, 2015, Vol. 103.

23. *Anti-Müllerian hormone exhibits a great variation in infertile women with different ovarian reserve patterns.* **Gorkem, Umit , et al.,** s.l. : Aust N Z J Obstet Gynaecol, 2017.

24. *Age-specific serum anti-Müllerian hormone values for 17,120 women presenting to fertility centers within the United States.* **Seifer, David, Baker, Valerie and Leader, Benjamin.** 2, s.l. : Fertility and Sterility, 2011, Vol. 95.

25. *Antimüllerian hormone in relation to tobacco and marijuana use and sources of indoor heating/cooking.* **White, Alexandra, et al.,** 3, s.l. : Fertility and Sterility, 2016, Vol. 106.

26. *Serum anti-Müllerian hormone and ovarian morphology assessed by magnetic resonance imaging in response to acupuncture and exercise in women with polycystic ovary syndrome: secondary analyses of a randomized controlled trial.* **Leonhardt, H, et al.,** 3, s.l. : Acta Obstet Gynecol Scand, 2015, Vol. 94.

27. *Efficacy of electroacupuncture in regulating the imbalance of AMH and FSH to improve follicle development and hyperandrogenism in PCOS rats.* **Shi, Yin, et al.,** s.l. : Biomedicine & Pharmacotherapy, 2019, Vol. 113.

28. *T-cell subsets (Th1 versus Th2).* **Romagnani, Sergio .** 1, s.l. : Ann Allergy Asthma Immunol, 2000, Vol. 85.

29. *The immune response during the luteal phase of the ovarian cycle: a Th2-type response?* **Faas, Marijke, et al.,** 5, s.l. : Fertility and Sterility, 2000, Vol. 74.

30. **Martini, Frederic.** *Fundamentals of Anatomy and Physiology.* Fourth. Upper

Saddle River : Prentice Hall Inc, 1998.

31. *Addition of dehydroepiandrosterone (DHEA) for poor-responder patients before and during IVF treatment improves the pregnancy rate: a randomized prospective study.* **Wiser, A, et al.,** s.l. : Human Reproduction, 2010.

32. *The use of coenzyme Q10 and DHEA during COH and IVF cycles in patients with decreased ovarian reserve (DOR).* **Gat, I, et al.,** 3, s.l. : Fertility and Sterility, 2015, Vol. 104.

33. *Update on the use of dehydroepiandrosterone supplementation among women with diminished ovarian function.* **Barad , David , Brill, Hyama and Gleicher, Norbert.** s.l. : J Assist Reprod Genet, 2007, Vol. 24.

34. *Effect of dehydroepiandrosterone on oocyte and embryo yields, embryo grade and cell number in IVF.* **Barad, David and Gleicher, Norbert.** 11, s.l. : Human Reproduction, 2006, Vol. 21.

35. *Control of GnRH neuronal activity by metabolic factors: the role of leptin and insulin.* **Gamba, Marcella and Pralong, Francois.** s.l. : Molecular and Cellular Endocrinology, 2006.

36. **Balen, Adam.** *Infertility in Practice.* Fourth Edition. Boca Raton : CRC Press, 2014.

37. *Low-Frequency Electro-Acupuncture and Physical Exercise Improve Metabolic Disturbances and Modulate Gene Expression in Adipose Tissue in Rats with Dihydrotestosterone-Induced Polycystic Ovary Syndrome.* **Mannerås, Louise, et al.,** 7, s.l. : Endocrinology, 2008, Vol. 149.

38. *Artificial Sweetener Use and One-Year Weight Change among Women.* **Stellman, Steven and Lawrence, Garfinkel.** s.l. : Preventive Medicine, 1986, Vol. 15.

39. **Tortora, Gerard and Derrickson, Bryan.** *Principles of Anatomy and Physiology.* Hoboken : John Wiley & Sons, 2014.

40. *Human female meiosis: what makes a good egg go bad?* **Hunt, P and Hassold, T.** 2, s.l. : Trends Genet, 2008, Vol. 24.

41. *Evidence for decreasing quality of semen during past 50 years.* **Carlsen, E, et al.,** s.l. : BMJ, 1992, Vol. 305.

42. **Kleeman, Julie and Yu, Harry.** *Oxford Chinese Dictionary.* Oxford : Oxford University Press, 2010.

43. **Maciocia, Giovanni.** *Obstetrics and Gynecology.* Edinburgh : Churchill Livingstone, 2011.

44. *Auricular acupuncture in the treatment of female infertility.* **Gerhard, I and Postneek, F.** s.l. : Gynecol. Endocrinol, 1992, Vol. 6.

45. *Energy intakes are higher during the luteal phase of ovulatory menstrual cycles.* **Barr, S, Janelle, K and Prior, J.** 1, s.l. : The American Journal of Clinical Nutrition, 1995, Vol. 61.

46. *'My fertility app made me too stressed to conceive'.* **Bearne, Suzanne .** s.l. : BBC, 6 April 2017.

47. **WHO.** *WHO laboratory manual for the examination and processing of human semen - Fifth edition.* Geneva : WHO, 2010.

48. *Temporal trends in sperm count: a systematic review and meta-regression analysis.* **Levine, H, et al.,** 6, s.l. : Hum Reprod Update, 2017, Vol. 23.

49. *Annual Patterns of Human Sperm Production and Semen Quality.* **Mortimer, D, et al.,** 1, s.l. : Archives of Andrology, 1983, Vol. 10.

50. *Clinical study on combined acupuncture with chinese medicine for infertility due to hydrosalpinx.* **Mi, Xiao-ying and Lin, Hong-bo.** 2, s.l. : Journal of Acupuncture and Tuina Science, 2012, Vol. 10.

51. *Effects of transcutaneous electrical acupoint stimulation on ovarian reserve of patients with diminished ovarian reserve in in vitro fertilization and embryo transfer cycles.* **Zheng, Y, et al.,** 12, s.l. : J Obstet Gynaecol Res, 2015, Vol. 41.

52. *Occupational factors and markers of ovarian reserve and response among women at a fertility centre.* **Mínguez-Alarcón, Lidia , et al.,** s.l. : BMJ, 2017, BMJ, pp. 1-6.

53. *Work schedule and physical factors in relation to fecundity in nurses.* **Gaskins, Audrey, et al.,** 2015, BMJ, pp. 1-7.

54. *Work schedule and physically demanding work in relation to menstrual function: the Nurses' Health Study 3.* **Lawson, C, et al.,** 2015, Scand J Work Environ

Health, pp. 194-203.

55. *Thromboprophylaxis improves the live birth rate in women with consecutive recurrent miscarriages and hereditary thrombophilia.* **Carp, H, Dolitzky, M and Inbal, A.** s.l. : Journal of Thrombosis and Haemostasis, 2003, Vol. 1.

56. *Interferon lambda protects the female reproductive tract against Zika virus infection.* **Caine, Elizabeth, et al.,** s.l. : Nature Communications, 2019, Vol. 10.

57. **Centres for Disease Control and Prevention.** *Zika Basics and How To Protect Yourself.* s.l. : U.S. Department of Health and Human Services, 2018.

58. **Centers for Disease Control and Prevention.** *Counseling Travelers on Zika Virus Risks.* Washington : U.S. Department of Health & Human Services, 2019.

59. *Genetic Considerations in Recurrent Pregnancy Loss.* **Hyde, Kassie and Schust, Danny.** 3, s.l. : Cold Spring Harb Perspect Med, 2015, Vol. 5.

60. *Prevalence of chromosomal abnormalities in couples with recurrent miscarriage.* **Elghezal, Hatem , et al.,** 3, s.l. : Fertility and Sterility, 2007, Vol. 88.

61. *Why natural killer cells are not enough: a further understanding of killer immunoglobulin-like receptor and human leukocyte antigen.* **Alecsandru, D and García-Velasco, J.** 6, s.l. : Fertility and Sterility, 2017, Vol. 107.

62. *Acupuncture on the Endometrial Morphology, the Serum Estradiol and Progesterone Levels, and the Expression of Endometrial Leukaemia-inhibitor Factor and Osteopontin in Rats.* **Fu, Houju, et al.,** s.l. : Evidence-Based Complementary and Alternative Medicine, 2011.

63. *Psychological Stress and the Human Immune System: A Meta-Analytic Study of 30 Years of Inquiry.* **Segerstrom , Suzanne and Miller, Gregory.** 4, s.l. : Psychological Bulletin, 2004, Vol. 130.

64. *Acupuncture and immune modulation.* **Kim, S and Bae, H.** s.l. : Autonomic Neuroscience, 2010, Vol. 157.

65. *Observation of a Flowing Duct in the Abdominal Wal lby Using Nano particles.* **Jang, H, et al.,** 3, s.l. : PLoS ONE, 2016, Vol. 11.

66. *The association between smoking and female infertility as influenced by cause of the infertility.* **Phipps, W, et al.,** 3, s.l. : Fertility and Sterility, 1987, Vol. 48.

67. *Smoking and reproduction.* **Stillman, R, Rosenberg, M and Sachs, B.** 4, s.l. : Fertility and Sterility, 1986, Vol. 46.

68. *Smoking Reduces Fecundity: A European Multicenter Study on Infertility and Subfecundity.* **Bolumar, F, Olsen, J and Boldsen, J.** 6, s.l. : American Journal of Epidemiology, 1996, Vol. 143.

69. *Prevention of chronic alcohol and nicotine-induced azospermia, sterility and decreased libido, by a novel tri-substituted benzoflavone moiety from Passiflora incarnata Linneaus in healthy male rats.* **Dhawan, Kamaldeep and Sharma, Anupam .** s.l. : Life Sciences, 2002, Vol. 71.

70. *The Insults of Illicit Drug Use on Male Fertility.* **Fronczak, C, Kim, E and Barqawi, A.** 4, s.l. : Journal of Andrology, 2012, Vol. 33.

71. *Chronic exposure to MDMA (ecstasy) increases DNA damage in sperm and alters testes histopathology in male rats.* **Barenys, M, et al.,** 1, s.l. : Toxicol Lett, 2000, Vol. 191.

72. *MDMA (ecstasy) delays pubertal development and alters sperm quality after developmental exposure in the rat.* **Barenys, M, et al.,** 2, s.l. : Toxicol Lett, 2010, Vol. 197.

73. *Exposure to cannabis alters the genetic profile of sperm.* **Murphy, Susan, et al.,** s.l. : Epigenetics, 2018.

74. *Environmental estrogen-like endocrine disrupting chemicals and breast cancer.* **Morgan, Marisa , et al.,** s.l. : Molecular and Cellular Endocrinology, 2017, Vol. 457.

75. *The effects of environmental hormones on reproduction.* **Danzo, B.** s.l. : CMLS, Cell. Mol. Life Sci, 1998, Vol. 54.

76. *Human infertility: are endocrine disruptors to blame?* **Marques-Pinto, A and Carvalho, D.** 3, s.l. : Endocr Connect, 2013, Vol. 2.

77. **Agency for Toxic Substances and Disease Registry (ATSDR).** *Toxicological Profile for DDT, DDE, DDD.* Atlanta : U.S. Department of Health and

Human Services, Public Health Service, 2002.

78. *Science linking environmental contaminant exposures with fertility and reproductive health impacts in the adult female.* **Mendola, Pauline , Messer, Lynne and Rappazzo, Kristen .** 2, s.l. : Fertility and Sterility, 2008, Vol. 89.

79. *Occurrence of pharmaceuticals and hormones in drinking water treated from surface waters.* **Vulliet, Emmanuelle , Cren-Olivé, Cécile and Grenier-Loustalot, Marie-Florence .** 1, s.l. : Environ Chem Lett, 2011, Vol. 9.

80. *Miscarriages associated with drinking water disinfection byproducts, study says.* **Betts, Kellyn.** s.l. : Environmental Science & Technology, 1998.

81. *Time To Pregnancy In Relation To Total Trihalomethane Levels In Tap Water.* **Mendola, P, et al.,** Vancouver : Presented at 14th Annual Meeting of International Society for Environmental Epidemiology, 2002.

82. *Environmental oestrogens, cosmetics and breast cancer.* **Darbre, P D.** 1, s.l. : Best Practice & Research Clinical Endocrinology & Metabolism, 2006, Vol. 20.

83. *Urinary and air phthalate concentrations and self-reported use of personal care products among minority pregnant women in New York city.* **Just, A, et al.,** s.l. : Journal of Exposure Science and Environmental Epidemiology, 2010, Vol. 20.

84. *Phthalate exposure among pregnant women in Jerusalem, Israel: results of a pilot study.* **Berman, T, et al.,** s.l. : Environment International, 2009, Vol. 35.

85. *Determination of bisphenol A concentrations in human biological fluids reveals significant early prenatal exposure.* **Ikezuki, Yumiko , et al.,** 11, s.l. : Human Reproduction, 2002, Vol. 17.

86. *Hormones and testis development and the possible adverse effects of environmental chemicals.* **Sharpe, Richard.** s.l. : Toxicology Letters, 2001, Vol. 120.

87. *Role of environmental estrogens in the deterioration of male factor fertility.* **Rozati, Roya , et al.,** 6, s.l. : Fertility and Sterility, 2002, Vol. 78.

88. *Urinary paracetamol and time-to-pregnancy.* **Smarr, Melissa, et al.,** s.l. : Human Reproduction, 2016.

89. *Intrauterine Exposure to Paracetamol and Aniline Impairs Female Reproductive Development by Reducing Follicle Reserves and Fertility.* **Holm, Jacob, et al.,** 1,

s.l. : Toxicological Sciences, 2016, Vol. 150.

90. *Paracetamol, aspirin and indomethacin display endocrine disrupting properties in the adult human testis in vitro.* **Albert, O, et al.,** 7, s.l. : Human Reproduction, 2013, Vol. 28.

91. *Paracetamol-associated luteinized unruptured follicle syndrome: effect on intrafollicular blood flow.* **Bourne, T, et al.,** s.l. : Ultrasound in Obstetrics and Gynecology, 1991.

92. *Polybrominated Diphenyl Ethers in Human Serum and Sperm Quality.* **Akutsu, K, et al.,** s.l. : Bull Environ Contam Toxicol, 2008, Vol. 80.

93. *House Dust Concentrations of Organophosphate Flame Retardants in Relation to Hormone Levels and Semen Quality Parameters.* **Meeker, John and Stapleton, Heather.** 3, s.l. : Environmental Health Perspectives, 2010, Vol. 118.

94. *In utero reproductive study in rats exposed to nonylphenol.* **Hossaini, Alireza , et al.,** s.l. : Reproductive Toxicology, 2001, Vol. 15.

95. *Emerging endocrine disrupters: perfluoroalkylated substances.* **Jensen, Allan and Leffers, Henrik .** s.l. : International Journal of Andrology, 2008, Vol. 31.

96. *Do Perfluoroalkyl Compounds Impair Human Semen Quality?* **Joensen, Ulla, et al.,** 6, s.l. : Environ Health Perspect, 2009, Vol. 117.

97. **National Collaborating Centre for Environmental Health.** *Potential human health effects of perfluorinated chemicals (PFCs).* British Columbia : British Columbia Centre for Disease Control, 2010.

98. *Is There a Critical Period for the Developmental Neurotoxicity of Low-Level Tobacco Smoke Exposure?* **Slotkin, Theodore, et al.,** s.l. : ToxSci Advance Access, 2016.

99. **BBC.** *Women's fertility delayed by pill.* London : BBC, 2004.

100. *Environmental chemical exposures and autism spectrum disorders: a review of the epidemiological evidence.* **Kalkbrenner, A, Schmidt, R and Penlesky, A.** 10, s.l. : Curr Probl Pediatr Adolesc Health Care, 2014, Vol. 44.

101. *Leptin and Pubertal Development.* **Mann, David and Plant, Tony.** 2, s.l. : Seminars in Reproductive Medicine, 2002, Vol. 20.

102. *Leptin and reproduction: a review.* **Moschos, Stergios , Chan, Jean and Mantzoros, Christos.** 3, s.l. : Fertility and Sterility, 2002, Vol. 77.

103. *Leptin in Reproduction.* **Caprio, Massimiliano , et al.,** 2, s.l. : Trends in Endocrinology & Metabolism, 2001, Vol. 12.

104. *The Distribution and Mechanism of Action of Ghrelin in the CNS Demonstrates a Novel Hypothalamic Circuit Regulating Energy Homeostasis.* **Cowley, Michael, et al.,** s.l. : Neuron, 2003, Vol. 37.

105. *Iron-Deficiency Anemia.* **Camaschella, Clara .** s.l. : The New England Journal of Medicine, 2015, Vol. 372.

106. *Weight loss results in significant improvement in pregnancy and ovulation rates in anovulatory obese women.* **Clark, A, et al.,** 10, s.l. : Human Reproduction, 1995, Vol. 10.

107. *Physical activity is negatively associated with antral follicle count.* **Bedrick, Bronwyn, et al.,** 3, s.l. : Fertility and Sterility, 2017, Vol. 107.

108. *International Committee for Monitoring Assisted Reproductive Technologies world report: Assisted Reproductive Technology 2008, 2009 and 2010.* **Dyer, S, et al.,** 2016, Human Reproduction.

109. *Air pollution combustion emissions: Characterization of causative agents and mechanisms associated with cancer, reproductive, and cardiovascular effects.* **Lewtas, Joellen .** 1-3, s.l. : Mutation Research/Reviews in Mutation Research, 2007, Vol. 636.

110. *The melatonin rhythm: both a clock and a calendar.* **Reiter, R.** 8, s.l. : Experientia, 1993, Vol. 49.

111. *Reactive oxygen species and oocyte aging: Role of superoxide, hydrogen peroxide, and hypochlorous acid.* **Goud, Anuradha, et al.,** 7, s.l. : Free Radical Biology and Medicine, 2008, Vol. 44.

112. *Antioxidant intake is associated with semen quality in healthy men.* **Eskenazi, B, et al.,** 4, s.l. : Human Reproduction, 2005, Vol. 20.

113. *Melatonin levels in follicular fluid as markers for IVF outcomes and predicting ovarian reserve.* **Tong, Jing , et al.,** 4, s.l. : Reproduction, 2017, Vol. 153.

114. *Revealing acupuncture meridian-like system by reactive oxygen species visualization.* **Guo, Jingke, et al.,** 6, s.l. : Bioscience Hypotheses, 2009, Vol. 2.

115. *Bonghan Circulatory System as an Extension of Acupuncture Meridians.* **Soh, Kwang-Sup .** 2, s.l. : J Acupunct Meridian Stud, 2009, Vol. 2.

116. *Influence of Shift Work on Early Reproductive Outcomes.* **Stocker, Linden, et al.,** 1, s.l. : Obstetrics & Gynecology, 2014, Vol. 124.

117. **Rochat De La Vallee, Elisabeth.** *A Study of Qi.* London : Monkey Press, 2013.

118. **Zhen, Li Shi.** *Pulse Diagnosis.* Brookline : Paradigm Pblications, 1985.

119. *Iron deficiency: new insights into diagnosis and treatment.* **Camaschella, Clara .** 13, s.l. : Hematology, 2015, Vol. 8.

120. *Risk-Based Questionnaires Fail to Detect Adolescent Iron Deficiency and Anemia.* **Sekhar, D, et al.,** s.l. : J Pediatr, 2017, Vol. 187.

121. **Cawley, Laurence .** *Fertility towns: Is there ever 'something in the water'?* London : BBC News, 2015.

122. **Maciocia, Giovanni.** *The Foundations of Chinee Medicine.* Edinburgh : Churchill Livingstone, 2005.

123. *Interactions between the Hypothalamic-Pituitary-Adrenal Axis and the Female Reproductive System: Clinical Implications.* **Chrousos, George, Torpy, David and Gold, Philip.** 3, s.l. : Annals of Internal Medicine, 1998, Vol. 129.

124. *Maternal sympathetic stress impairs follicular development and puberty of the offspring.* **Barra, R, et al.,** 2, s.l. : Reproduction, 2014, Vol. 148.

125. *Efficacy of Traditional Chinese Herbal Medicine in the management of female infertility: a systematic review.* **Ried, K and Stuart, K.** 6, s.l. : Complement Ther Med, 2011, Vol. 19.

126. *Occupational factors and markers of ovarian reserve and response among women at a fertility centre.* **Mínguez-Alarcón, Lidia , et al.,** s.l. : Occup Environ Med, 2017.

127. *The more, the better? the impact of sleep on IVF outcomes.* **Park, I, et al.,** 3, s.l. : Fertility and Sterility, 2013, Vol. 100.

128. *Is Sedentary Lifestyle Associated With Testicular Function? A Cross-Sectional Study of 1,210 Men.* **Priskorn, Lærke, et al.,** 2016, American Journal of Epidemiology, pp. 284-294.

129. *Auricular Acupuncture in the Treatment of Cocaine/Crack Abuse: A Review of the Efficacy, the Use of the National Acupuncture Detoxification Association Protocol, and the Selection of Sham Points.* **D'Alberto, Attilio.** 6, s.l. : The Journal of Alternative and Complementary Medicine, 2004, Vol. 10.

130. *Understanding Cocaine Addiction According to Chinese Medicine Theory.* **D'Alberto, Attilio.** 1, s.l. : EJOM, 2015, Vol. 8.

131. *Changes in Serum Leptin and Beta Endorphin Levels with Weight Loss by Electroacupuncture and Diet Restriction in Obesity Treatment.* **Cabıoğlu , Mehmet Tuğrul and Ergene , Neyhan .** 1, s.l. : The American Journal of Chinese Medicine, 2006, Vol. 34.

132. *Copper regulates cyclic-AMP-dependent lipolysis.* **Krishnamoorthy, Lakshmi , et al.,** s.l. : Nature Chemical Biology, 2016, Vol. 12.

133. *The Histochemistry of Complex Carbohydrates in the Ovarian Follicles of Adult Mice.* **Tadano, Y and Yamada, K.** s.l. : Histochemistry, 1978, Vol. 57.

134. *Human FSH isoforms: carbohydrate complexity as determinant of in-vitro bioactivity.* **Creus, Silvina , et al.,** s.l. : Molecular and Cellular Endocrinology, 2001, Vol. 174.

135. *Acupuncture for Chronic Pain: Update of an Individual Patient Data Meta-Analysis.* **Vickers, Andrew, et al.,** 5, s.l. : The Journal of Pain, 2017, Vol. 19.

136. *Reduction of the incidence of sperm DNA fragmentation by oral antioxidant treatment.* **Greco, E, et al.,** 3, s.l. : J Androl, 2005, Vol. 26.

137. *Effects of folic acid and zinc sulfate on male factor subfertility: a double-blind, randomized, placebo-controlled trial.* **Wong, Wai Yee, et al.,** 3, s.l. : Fertility and Sterility, 2002, Vol. 77.

138. *Effects of Parenteral Lipid Emulsions With Different Fatty Acid Composition on Immune Cell Functions In Vitro.* **Granato, D.** 2000, Journal of Parenteral and Enteral Nutritio, pp. 113-8.

139. *The Effect of Acupuncture on Psychosocial Outcomes for Women Experiencing Infertility: A Pilot Randomized Controlled Trial.* **Smith, Caroline, et al.,** 10, s.l. : J Altern Complement Med, 2011, Vol. 17.

140. *Parental olfactory experience influences behavior and neural structure in subsequent generations.* **Dias, Brian and Ressler, Kerry.** 1, s.l. : Nature Neuroscience, 2014, Vol. 17.

141. *Coping and the ineffectiveness of coping influence the outcome of in vitro fertilization through stress responses.* **Demyttenaere, K, et al.,** 6, s.l. : Psychoneuroendocrinology, 1992, Vol. 17.

142. *Relationship between hair and salivary cortisol and pregnancy in women undergoing IVF.* **Massey, A, et al.,** s.l. : Psychoneuroendocrinology, 2016, Vol. 74.

143. *Psychological interactions with infertility among women.* **Cwikel, J, Gidron, Y and Sheiner, E.** s.l. : European Journal of Obstetrics & Gynecology and Reproductive Biology, 2004, Vol. 117.

144. *Preconception stress increases the risk of infertility: results from a couple-based prospective cohort study—the LIFE study.* **Lynch, C, et al.,** 5, s.l. : Human Reproduction, 2014, Vol. 29.

145. *Immunological changes and stress are associated with different implantation rates in patients undergoing in vitro fertilization–embryo transfer.* **Gallinelli, Andrea , et al.,** 1, s.l. : Fertility and Sterility, 2001, Vol. 76.

146. *Changes in serum cortisol and prolactin associated with acupuncture during controlled ovarian hyperstimulation in women undergoing in vitro fertilization-embryo transfer treatment.* **Magarelli, P, Cridennda, D and Cohen, M.** 6, s.l. : Fertility and Sterility, 2009, Vol. 92.

147. *Coping style and depress!on level influence outcome in in vitro fertilization.* **Demyttenaere, Koen , et al.,** 6, s.l. : Fertility and Sterility, 1998, Vol. 69.

148. *Consumer product exposures associated with urinary phthalate levels in pregnant women.* **Buckley, Jessie, et al.,** s.l. : Journal of Exposure Science and Environmental Epidemiology, 2012, Vol. 22.

149. **WHO.** *Ambient air pollution: A global assessment of exposure and burden of*

disease. Geneva : World Health Organisation, 2016.

150. *The biological effects of carbon monoxide on the pregnant woman, fetus, and newborn infant* . **Longo, Lawrence.** 1977, American Journal of Obstetrics and Gynecology, pp. 69-103.

151. *B vitamins attenuate the epigenetic effects of ambient fine particles in a pilot human intervention trial.* **Zhong, Jia, et al.,** 2017, Proceedings of the National Academy of Sciences, pp. 3503-3508.

152. *Placental Mitochondrial DNA Content and Particulate Air Pollution during in Utero Life.* **Janssen, Bram, et al.,** 2012, Environmental Health Perspectives, pp. 1346-1352.

153. *Chronic exposure to fine particulate matter emitted by traffic affects reproductive and fetal outcomes in mice.* **Veras, Mariana, et al.,** 5, s.l. : Environmental Research, 2009, Vol. 109.

154. *Cadmium toxicity: a possible cause of male infertility in Nigeria.* **Akinloye, Oluyemi, et al.,** s.l. : Society for Biology of Reproduction, 2006, Reproductive Biology, pp. 17-30.

155. *Cadmium Determination in Mexican-Produced Tobacco.* **Saldivar De R, Liliana, et al.,** 1991, Environmental Research, Vol. 55, pp. 91-96.

156. *Cadmium: Toxic effects on the reproductive system and the embryo.* **Thompson, Jennifer and Bannigan, John.** 2008, Reproductive Toxicology, pp. 304-315.

157. *Exposure to Lead and Male Fertility.* **Sallmen, Markku.** 3, s.l. : International Journal of Occupational Medicine and Environmental Health, 2001, Vol. 14.

158. *Impact of heavy metals on the female reproductive system.* **Rzymski, Piotr , et al.,** 2, s.l. : Annals of Agricultural and Environmental Medicine, 2015, Vol. 22.

159. *Hong Kong male subfertility links to mercury in human hair and fish.* **Dickman, M, Leung, C and Leong, M.** s.l. : The Science of the Total Environment, 1998, Vol. 214.

160. *Hong Kong male subfertility links to mercury in human hair and fish* **Dickman, M, Leung, C and Leong, M.** 1998, The Science of the Total Environment , pp. 165-174.

161. *Low dose mercury toxicity and human health.* **Zahir, Farhana, et al.,** 2, s.l. : Environmental Toxicology and Pharmacology, 2005, Vol. 20.

162. *Effect of cell phone usage on semen analysis in men attending infertility clinic: an observational study.* **Agarwal, Ashok , et al.,** 2008, Fertility and Sterility, pp. 124–128.

163. *Effects of radiofrequency electromagnetic waves (RF-EMW) from cellular phones on human ejaculated semen: an in vitro pilot study.* **Agarwal, Ashok , et al.,** 2009, Fertility and Sterility, pp. 1318–1325.

164. *Alterations in TSH and Thyroid Hormones following Mobile Phone Use.* **Mortavazi, Seyed , et al.,** 4, s.l. : Oman Med J, 2009, Vol. 24.

165. *Use of laptop computers connected to internet through Wi-Fi decreases human sperm motility and increases sperm DNA fragmentation.* **Avendaño, Conrado , et al.,** 2012, Fertility and Sterility, pp. 39–45.

166. *Study on Microwave Absorbing of Tourmaline and Dravite/ZnO Complex Powders.* **Zhang, Xiaohui and Ma, Hongwen.** s.l. : Advanced Materials Research Vols, 2014.

167. *Paracetamol, Aspirin, and Indomethacin Induce Endocrine Disturbances in the Human Fetal Testis Capable of Interfering With Testicular Descent.* **Mazaud-Guittot, Séverine , et al.,** s.l. : J Clin Endocrinol Metab, 2013, Vol. 98.

168. *Prostaglandin E2 involvement in mammalian female fertility: ovulation, fertilization, embryo development and early implantation.* **Niringiyumukiza, Jean, Cai, Hongcai and Xiang, Wenpei .** 43, s.l. : Reproductive Biology and Endocrinology, 2018, Vol. 16.

169. *Effects of Some Non Steroidal Anti-Inflammatory Drugs on Ovulation in Women with Mild Musculoskeletal Pain.* **Salman, S, Sherif , B and Al-Zohyri, A.** s.l. : Annals of the Rheumatic Diseases, 2015, Vol. 74.

170. *Nonsteroidal Anti-Inflammatory Drugs Alter Body Temperature and Suppress Melatonin in Humans.* **Murphy, P, Myers, B and Badia, P.** 1, s.l. : Physiology & Behavior, 1996, Vol. 59.

171. *Non-pharmacological treatments for pain relief: TENS and acupuncture.* **Coutaux, Anne .** 6, s.l. : Joint Bone Spine, 2017, Vol. 84.

172. *Maternal Use of Selective Serotonin Reuptake Inhibitors and Risk of Congenital Malformations.* **Wogelius, Pia , et al.,** 2006, Epidemiology, pp. 701-4.

173. *Antidepressant Use During Pregnancy and the Risk of Autism Spectrum Disorder in Children.* **Boukhris, Takoua, et al.,** 2015, JAMA Pediatrics, pp. E1-8.

174. *Antidepressant use during pregnancy and the risk of major congenital malformations in a cohort of depressed pregnant women: an updated analysis of the Quebec Pregnancy Cohort.* **Bérard, Anick , Zhao, Jin-Ping and Sheehy, Odile** . 2017, BMJ, pp. 1-13.

175. *Association of Selective Serotonin Reuptake Inhibitor Exposure During Pregnancy With Speech, Scholastic, and Motor Disorders in Offspring.* **Brown, Alan, et al.,** 2016, JAMA Psychiatry, pp. E1-8.

176. *Are Selective Serotonin Reuptake Inhibitors Cardiac Teratogens? Echocardiographic Screening of Newborns with Persistent Heart Murmur.* **Merlob, Paul , et al.,** 2009, Birth Defects Research, pp. 837– 841.

177. *First Trimester Exposure to Paroxetine and Risk of Cardiac Malformations in Infants: The Importance of Dosage.* **Bérard, Anick, et al.,** 2007, Birth Defects Research, pp. 18-27.

178. *First-Trimester Use of Paroxetine and Congenital Heart Defects: A Population-Based Case-Control Study.* **Bakker, Marian, et al.,** 2010, Birth Defects Research, pp. 94-100.

179. *Major Congenital Malformations Following Prenatal Exposure to Serotonin Reuptake Inhibitors and Benzodiazepines Using Population-Based Health Data.* **Oberlander, Tim, et al.,** 2008, Birth Defects Research, pp. 68-76.

180. *Paroxetine and Congenital Malformations: Meta-Analysis and Consideration of Potential Confounding Factors.* **Bar-Oz, Benjamin , et al.,** 2007, Clinical Therapeutics, pp. 918-926.

181. *Selective Serotonin Reuptake Inhibitor (SSRI) Antidepressants in Pregnancy and Congenital Anomalies: Analysis of Linked Databases in Wales, Norway and Funen, Denmark.* **Jordan, Sue , et al.,** 2016, Plos One, pp. 1-26.

182. *Selective serotonin reuptake inhibitors and adverse pregnancy outcomes.* **Wen, Shi Wu, et al.,** 2006, American Journal of Obstetrics and Gynecology, pp.

961-966.

183. *Effect of Acupressure, Acupuncture and Moxibustion in Women With Pregnancy-Related Anxiety and Previous Depression: A Preliminary Study.* **Suzuki, Shunji and Tobe, Chiharu**. 6, s.l. : J Clin Med Res, 2017, Vol. 9.

184. *Malformation risks of antiepileptic drugs in pregnancy: a prospective study from the UK Epilepsy and Pregnancy Register.* **Morrow, J, et al.,** s.l. : J Neurol Neurosurg Psychiatry, 2006, Vol. 77.

185. *Treatment for epilepsy in pregnancy: neurodevelopmental outcomes in the child (Review).* **Bromley, R, et al.,** 10, s.l. : The Cochrane Library, 2014.

186. *Exposition in utero à l'acide valproïque et aux autres traitements de l'épilepsie et des troubles bipolaires et risque de malformations congénitales majeures (MCM) en France.* **Raguideau, F, et al.,** 2017, Synthèse.

187. *Prenatal Valproate Exposure and Risk of Autism Spectrum Disorders and Childhood Autism.* **Christensen, Jakob , et al.,** 16, s.l. : JAMA, 2013, Vol. 309.

188. **Pitchford, Paul.** *Healing with Whole Foods.* Third. Berkeley : North Atlantic Books, 2002.

189. *Lifestyle factors and reproductive health: taking control of your fertility.* **Sharma, Rakesh , et al.,** 66, s.l. : Reprod Biol Endocrinol, 2013, Vol. 11.

190. *Caffeinated Beverages And Decreased Fertility.* **Wilcox, Allen, Weinberg, Clarice and Baird, Donna .** s.l. : The Lancet, 1988, Vol. 332.

191. **Mindell, Earl and Mundis, Hester.** *Eael Mindell's New Vitamin Bible.* New York : Hachette Book Group, 2011.

192. *Association of vitamin D intake and serum levels with fertility: results from the Lifestyle and Fertility Study.* **Fung, June, et al.,** 2017, Fertility & Sterility.

193. *Opiate-like effects of sugar on gene expression in reward areas of the rat brain.* **Spangler, Rudolph , et al.,** 2, s.l. : Molecular Brain Research, 2004, Vol. 124.

194. *Relationship of omega-3 and omega-6 fatty acids with semen characteristics, and anti-oxidant status of seminal plasma: a comparison between fertile and infertile men.* **Safarinejad, M, et al.,** 1, s.l. : Clin Nutr, 2010, Vol. 29.

195. *Processed Meat Intake Is Unfavorably and Fish Intake Favorably Associated with*

Semen Quality Indicators among Men Attending a Fertility Clinic. **Afeiche, Myriam, et al.**, s.l. : The Journal of Nutrition, 2014, Vol. 144.

196. **Development Initiatives, 2017.** *Global Nutrition Report 2017.* Bristol : Global Nutrition Report, 2017.

197. **Brownstein, David.** *Iodine: Why You Need It, Why You Can't Live Without It.* West Bloomfield : Medical Alternative Press, 2014.

198. *Gender Differences in Coffee Consumption and Its Effects in Young People.* **Demura, Shinichi, et al.**, 7, s.l. : Food and Nutrition Sciences, 2013, Vol. 4.

199. *Coffee and caffeine intake and male infertility: a systematic review.* **Ricci, Elena, et al.**, 37, s.l. : Nutrition Journal, 2017, Vol. 16.

200. *Calcium Signals for Egg Activation in Mammals.* **Miyazaki, Shunichi and Ito, Masahiko.** s.l. : J Pharmacol Sci, 2006, Vol. 100.

201. *Does moderate alcohol consumption affect fertility? Follow up study among couples planning first pregnancy.* **Jensen, Tina, et al.**, s.l. : BMJ, 1998, Vol. 317.

202. *Habitual alcohol consumption associated with reduced semen quality and changes in reproductive hormones; a cross-sectional study among 1221 young Danish men.* **Jensen, Tina, et al.**, s.l. : BMJ Open, 2014, Vol. 4.

203. *Does alcohol have any effect on male reproductive function? A review of literature.* **La Vignera, Sandro, et al.**, 2, s.l. : Asian J Androl, 2013, Vol. 15.

204. *Comparison of the antiobesity effects of the protopanaxadiol- and protopanaxatriol-type saponins of red ginseng.* **Kim, Ji Hyun, et al.**, s.l. : Phytotherapy Research, 2009, Vol. 23.

205. *Ly6C^{hi} Monocytes Provide a Link between Antibiotic-Induced Changes in Gut Microbiota and Adult Hippocampal Neurogenesis.* **Möhle, Luisa, et al.**, 9, s.l. : Cell Reports, 2016, Vol. 15.

206. *Behavior of Some Solid Food Simulants in Contact with Several Plastics Used in Microwave Ovens.* **Nerín, Cristina and Acosta, Domingo.** 25, s.l. : J. Agric. Food Chem, 2002, Vol. 50.

207. *Microwave Heating Causes Rapid Degradation of Antioxidants in Polypropylene Packaging, Leading to Greatly Increased Specific Migration to Food Simulants As*

Shown by ESI-MS and GC-MS. **Alin, Jonas and Hakkarainen, Minna .** 10, s.l. : J. Agric. Food Chem, 2011, Vol. 59.

208. *Hazards of microwave cooking: direct thermal damage to the pharynx and larynx.* **Ford, G and Horrocks, C.** s.l. : The Journal of Laryngology & Otology, 1994, Vol. 108.

209. *Thermal injury to the upper aerodigestive tract after microwave heating of food.* **Offer, G, Nanan, D and Marshall, J.** s.l. : Journal of Accident and Emergency Medicine, 1995, Vol. 12.

210. *The pros and cons of phytoestrogens.* **Patisaul, Heather and Jefferson, Wendy.** 4, s.l. : Frontiers in Neuroendocrinology, 2010, Vol. 31.

211. *A specific breeding problem of sheep on subterranean clover pastures in Western Australia.* **Bennetts, H, Uuderwood, E and Shier, F.** 1, s.l. : The Australian Veterinary Journal, 1946, Vol. 22.

212. *Estimated Asian adult soy protein and isoflavone intakes.* **Messina, M, Nagata, C and Wu, A.** 1, s.l. : Nutrition and Cancer, 2006, Vol. 55.

213. *International Committee for Monitoring Assisted Reproductive Technologies world report: Assisted Reproductive Technology 2008, 2009 and 2010.* **Dyer, S, et al.,** s.l. : Human Reproduction, 2016.

214. *Effects of soy protein and isoflavones on circulating hormone concentrations in pre- and post-menopausal women: a systematic review and meta-analysis.* **Hooper, L, et al.,** 4, s.l. : Human Reproduction Update, 2009, Vol. 15.

215. *Soy, phyto-oestrogens and male reproductive function: a review.* **Cederroth, Christopher, et al.,** s.l. : International Journal of Andrology, 2010, Vol. 33.

216. *Effect of polyphenols on production of steroid hormones from human adrenocortical NCI-H295R cells.* **Hasegawa, E, et al.,** 2, s.l. : Biol Pharm Bull, 2013, Vol. 36.

217. *The Flavonoid Apigenin Is a Progesterone Receptor Modulator with In Vivo Activity in the Uterus.* **Dean, Matthew, et al.,** s.l. : Hormones and Cancer, 2018.

218. *Apigenin: A Promising Molecule for Cancer Prevention.* **Shukla, Sanjeev and Gupta, Sanjay .** 6, s.l. : Pharm Res, 2010, Vol. 27.

219. *Modulation of Androgen and Progesterone Receptors by Phytochemicals in Breast Cancer Cell Lines.* **Rosenberg, Rachel, et al.,** s.l. : Biochemical and Biophysical Research Communications, 1998, Vol. 248.

220. *Dietary flavonoid sources in Australian adults.* **Somerset, S and Johannot, L.** 4, s.l. : Nutr Cancer, 2008, Vol. 60.

221. *Effect of oral administration of Tribulus terrestris extract on semen quality and body fat index of infertile men.* **Salgado, R, et al.,** s.l. : Andrologia, 2016.

222. *Effects of Apigenin on Steroidogenesis and Steroidogenic Acute Regulatory Gene Expression in Mouse Leydig Cells.* **Li, Wei, et al.,** 3, s.l. : The Journal of Nutritional Biochemistry, 2011, Vol. 22.

223. *Effects of Some Non Steroidal Anti-inflammatory Drugs on Ovulation in Women with Mild Musculoskeletal Pain (A Clinical Study).* **Sherif, B, Al-Zohyri, A and Shihab, S.** 4, s.l. : Journal of Pharmacy and Biological Sciences, 2014, Vol. 9.

224. *Prevention of Oxidative Stress Injury to Sperm.* **Agarwal, A, Prabakaran, S and Said, T.** 6, s.l. : Journal of Andrology, 2005, Vol. 26.

225. *Lipid Peroxidation and Human Sperm Motility: Protective Role of Vitamin E.* **Suleiman, S, et al.,** 5, s.l. : Journal of Andrology, 1996, Vol. 17.

226. *Vitex agnus castus A Systematic Review of Adverse Events.* **Daniele, Claudia , et al.,** 4, s.l. : Drug Safety, 2005, Vol. 28.

227. *Therapeutic Effect of Vitex Agnus Castus in Patients with Premenstrual Syndrome.* **Zamani, Mehrangiz , Neghab, Nosrat and Torabian, Saadat .** 2, s.l. : Acta Medica Iranica, 2012, Vol. 50.

228. *Treatment of premenstrual tension syndrome with Vitex agnus castus. Controlled, double-blind study versus pyridoxine.* **Lauritzen, C, et al.,** 3, s.l. : Phytomedicine, 1997, Vol. 4.

229. *Vitex agnus-castus Extracts for Female Reproductive Disorders: A Systematic Review of Clinical Trials.* **Diana van Die, M, et al.,** s.l. : Planta Med, 2013, Vol. 79.

230. *Die Wirksamkeit des Komplexmittels Phyto-Hypophyson L bei weiblicher, hormonell bedingter Sterilitat.* **Bergmann, J, et al.,** s.l. : Forsch

KomplementaÈrmed Klass Naturheilkd, 2007, Vol. 7.

231. **Brewer, Sarah.** *The Essential Guide to Vitamins, Minerals and Herbal Supplements.* London : Right Way, 2010.

232. *Role of reactive oxygen species in male infertility.* **Sharma, Rakesh and Agarwal, Ashok .** 6, s.l. : Urology, 1996, Vol. 48.

233. *Beta-carotene, vitamin A and carrier proteins in thyroid diseases.* **Aktuna, D, et al.,** s.l. : Acta Medica Austriaca, 1993, Vol. 20.

234. *The Combination of N-Acetyl Cysteine, Alpha-Lipoic Acid, and Bromelain Shows High Anti-Inflammatory Properties in Novel In Vivo and In Vitro Models of Endometriosis.* **Agostinis, C, et al.,** s.l. : Mediators of Inflammation, 2015.

235. *Properties and Therapeutic Application of Bromelain: A Review.* **Pavan, Rajendra, et al.,** s.l. : Biotechnology Research International, 2012.

236. *In vivo and in vitro Effects of Bromelain on PGE2 and SP Concentrations in the Inflammatory Exudate in Rats.* **Gaspani, Leda, et al.,** s.l. : Pharmacology, 2002, Vol. 65.

237. *Effect of Chlorella vulgaris on Immune-enhancement and Cytokine Production in vivo and in vitro.* **An, Hyo-Jin, et al.,** 5, s.l. : Food Science and Biotechnology, 2008, Vol. 17.

238. *Dietary chromium deficiency effect on sperm count and fertility in rats.* **Anderson, Richard and Polansky, Marilyn.** 1, s.l. : Biological Trace Element Research, 1981, Vol. 3.

239. *Maternal vitamin A supplementation in relation to selected birth defects.* **Werler, Martha, et al.,** s.l. : Teratology, 1990, Vol. 42.

240. *Polyunsaturated Fatty Acids in Male and Female Reproduction.* **Wathes, Claire , Abayasekara, Robert and Aitken, John .** s.l. : Bioology of Reproduction, 2007, Vol. 77.

241. *Coenzyme Q10 restores oocyte mitochondrial function and fertility during reproductive aging.* **Ben-Meir, Assaf , et al.,** s.l. : Aging Cell, 2015, Vol. 14.

242. **Bensky, Dan , et al.,** *Materia Medica: Chinese Herbal Medicine.* Seattle : Eastland Press, 2004.

243. *The effects of combined conventional treatment, oral antioxidants and essential fatty acids on sperm biology in subfertile men.* **Comhaire, F, et al.,** 3, s.l. : Prostaglandins Leukot Essent Fatty Acids, 2000, Vol. 63.

244. *Long-chain n-3 PUFA: plant v. marine sources.* **Williams, Christine and Burdge, Graham .** s.l. : Proceedings of the Nutrition Society, 2006, Vol. 65.

245. *Dehydroepiandrosterone (DHEA) reduces embryo aneuploidy: direct evidence from preimplantation genetic screening (PGS).* **Gleicher, Norbert , Weghofer, Andrea and Barad, David.** s.l. : Reproductive Biology and Endocrinology, 2010, Vol. 8.

246. *Effects of isoliquiritigenin on ovarian antral follicle growth and steroidogenesis.* **Mahalingam, S, et al.,** s.l. : Reprod Toxicol, 2016.

247. **Viswanathan, M, Treiman, K and Doto, J.** *Folic Acid Supplementation: An Evidence Review for the U.S. Preventive Services Task Force.* s.l. : Agency for Healthcare Research and Quality (US), 2017.

248. *Preconceptional use of folic acid and knowledge about folic acid among low-income pregnant women in Korea.* **Kim, Jihyun , et al.,** 3, s.l. : Nutr Res Pract, 2017, Vol. 11.

249. *Association Between Maternal Use of Folic Acid Supplements and Risk of Autism Spectrum Disorders in Children.* **Suren, Pal, et al.,** 6, s.l. : JAMA, 2013, Vol. 309.

250. *Folic Acid Supplements in Pregnancy and Severe Language Delay in Children.* **Roth, Christine , et al.,** 14, s.l. : JAMA, 2011, Vol. 306.

251. **Fulder, Stephen.** *The Book of Ginseng.* Rochester : Healing Arts Press, 1980.

252. *Leptin Resistance and Obesity.* **Enriori, Pablo, et al.,** s.l. : Obseity, 2006, Vol. 14.

253. *Central Inflammation and Leptin Resistance Are Attenuated by Ginsenoside Rb1 Treatment in Obese Mice Fed a High-Fat Diet.* **Wu, Yizhen, et al.,** 3, s.l. : PLOS ONE, 2014, Vol. 9.

254. *Traditional Asian folklore medicines in sexual health.* **Lim Huat Chye, Peter .** 3, s.l. : Indian Journal of Urology, 2006, Vol. 22.

255. *L-Arginine Stimulation of Human Sperm Motility in vitro.* **Keller, D and Polakoski, K.** 2, s.l. : Biology of Reproduction, 1975, Vol. 13.

256. *Nitric oxide synthase and nitrite production in human spermatozoa: evidence that endogenous nitric oxide is beneficial to sperm motility.* **Lewis, S, et al.,** 11, s.l. : Molecular Human Reproduction, 1996, Vol. 2.

257. *Adjuvant L-arginine treatment for in-vitro fertilization in poor responder patients.* **Battaglia, Cesare , et al.,** 7, s.l. : Human Reproduction, 1999, Vol. 14.

258. *Lycopene and male infertility.* **Durairajanayaga, Damayanthi , et al.,** s.l. : Asian Journal of Andrology, 2-14, Vol. 16.

259. *Lycopene therapy in idiopathic male infertility – a preliminary report.* **Gupta, N and Kumar, R.** s.l. : International Urology and Nephrology, 2002, Vol. 34.

260. *Lepidium meyenii (Maca) enhances the serum levels of luteinising hormone in female rats.* **Uchiyama, Fumiaki , et al.,** 2, s.l. : Journal of Ethnopharmacology, 2014, Vol. 151.

261. *The Functions of Corticosteroid-Binding Globulin and Sex Hormone-Binding Globulin: Recent Advances.* **Rosner, W.** 1, s.l. : Endocrine Reviews, 1990, Vol. 11.

262. *Randomized, double blind placebo-controlled trial: effects of Myo-inositol on ovarian function and metabolic factors in women with PCOS.* **Gerli, S, et al.,** s.l. : European Review for Medical and Pharmacological Sciences, 2007, Vol. 11.

263. *Effects of Myo-Inositol supplementation on oocyte's quality in PCOS patients: a double blind trial.* **Ciotta, L, et al.,** s.l. : European Review for Medical and Pharmacological Sciences, 2011, Vol. 15.

264. *Myo-inositol in patients with polycystic ovary syndrome: A novel method for ovulation induction.* **Papaleo, Enrico, et al.,** s.l. : Gynecological Endocrinology, 2007, Vol. 23.

265. *Effects of myo-inositol in women with PCOS: a systematic review of randomized controlled trials, Gynecological Endocrinology.* **Unfer, V, et al.,** 7, s.l. : Gynecological Endocrinology, 2012, Vol. 28.

266. **Royal Pharmaceutical Society.** *British National Formulary - 76.* London :

BNF, 2018.

267. *Dietary pyrroloquinoline quinone (PQQ) alters indicators of inflammation and mitochondrial-related metabolism in human subjects.* **Harris, Calliandra, et al.,** 12, s.l. : The Journal of Nutritional Biochemistry, 2013, Vol. 24.

268. *The autoimmune bases of infertility and pregnancy loss.* **Carp, Howard, Selmi, Carlo and Shoenfeld, Yehuda .** 2-3, s.l. : Journal of Autoimmunity, 2012, Vol. 38.

269. *Effect of Spirulina on the Secretion of Cytokines from Peripheral Blood Mononuclear Cells.* **Mao, T, Gershwin, M and Van de Water, J.** 3, s.l. : Journal of Medicinal Food, 2000, Vol. 3.

270. *Potential health benefits of spirulina microalgae.* **Capelli, Bob and Cysewski, Gerald.** 2, s.l. : Nutra Foods, 2010, Vol. 9.

271. *Inhibitory effect of curcumin on angiogenesis in ectopic endometrium of rats with experimental endometriosis.* **Zhang, Y, et al.,** 1, s.l. : Int J Mol Med, 2011, Vol. 27.

272. *Curcumin inhibits endometriosis endometrial cells by reducing estradiol production.* **Zhang, Y, et al.,** 5, s.l. : Iran J Reprod Med, 2013, Vol. 11.

273. *Novel dietary supplement association reduces symptoms in endometriosis patients.* **Signorile, P, Viceconte, R and Baldi, A.** 8, s.l. : J Cell Physiol, 2018, Vol. 233.

274. *Can Herbal Medicines Improve Cellular Immunity Patterns in Endometriosis?* **Harris, T and Vlass, A.** 2, s.l. : Medicinal & Aromatic Plants, 2015, Vol. 4.

275. *Effect of Ubiquinol on Serum Reproductive Hormones of Amenorrhic Patients.* **Thakur, A, et al.,** s.l. : Ind J Clin Biochem, 2015.

276. *Ascorbic acid protects against endogenous oxidative DNA damage in human sperm.* **Fraga, C, et al.,** s.l. : Proc. Nati. Acad. Sci., 1991, Vol. 88.

277. *Vitamin D in cutaneous carcinogenesis: Part I.* **Tang, Jean, et al.,** 5, s.l. : J Am Acad Dermatol, 2012, Vol. 67.

278. *Zinc, copper and selenium in reproduction.* **Bedwal, R and Bahuguna, A.** 7, s.l. : Experientia, 1994, Vol. 50.

279. *Effect of Zinc Administration on Plasma Testosterone, Dihydrotestosterone,*

and Sperm Count. **Netter, A, Nahoul, K and Hartoma, R.** s.l. : Journal of Reproductive Systems, 1981, Vol. 7.

280. *Effect of zinc on human sperm motility and the acrosome reaction.* **Riffo, M, Leiva, S and Astudillo, J.** s.l. : International Journal of Andrology, 1992, Vol. 15.

281. *The zinc spark is an inorganic signature of human egg activation.* **Duncan, Francesca, et al.,** s.l. : Nature, 2016.

282. **Impey, L and Child, T.** *Obstetrics & Gynaecology.* Chichester : John Wiley & Sons, 2012.

283. *Prior to Conception: The Role of an Acupuncture Protocol in Improving Women's Reproductive Functioning Assessed by a Pilot Pragmatic Randomised Controlled Trial.* **Cochrane, S, et al.,** s.l. : Evid Based Complement Alternat Med, 2016.

284. *Complete mapping of the tattoos of the 5300-year-old Tyrolean Iceman.* **Samadelli, Marco , et al.,** 5, s.l. : Journal of Cultural Heritage, 2015, Vol. 16.

285. **Cheng, Xinnong.** *Chinese Acupuncture and Moxibustion.* Beijing : Foreign Languages Press, 1999.

286. *Safety of Acupuncture: Results of a Prospective Observational Study with 229,230 Patients and Introduction of a Medical Information and Consent Form.* **Witt, Claudia, et al.,** s.l. : Forsch Komplementmed, 2009, Vol. 16.

287. *The Primo Vascular System as a New Anatomical System.* **Stefanov, Miroslav , et al.,** 6, s.l. : Journal of Acupuncture and Meridian Studies, 2013, Vol. 6.

288. *Structure and Distribution of an Unrecognized Interstitium in Human Tissues.* **Benias, Petros, et al.,** s.l. : Nature, 2018.

289. *Effect of Acupuncture on Endometrial Angiogenesis and Uterus Dendritic Cells in COH Rats during Peri-Implantation Period.* **Dong, Haoxu, et al.,** s.l. : Evidence-Based Complementary and Alternative Medicine, 2017.

290. *Electroacupuncture for reproductive hormone levels in patients with diminished ovarian reserve: a prospective observational study.* **Wang, Yang , et al.,** s.l. : Acupuncture in Medicine, 2016.

291. *Changes in Levels of Serum Insulin, C-Peptide and Glucose after*

Electroacupuncture and Diet Therapy in Obese Women. **Cabıoglu , Mehmet and Ergene, Neyhan .** 3, s.l. : The American Journal of Chinese Medicine, 2006, Vol. 34.

292. *Effect of acupuncture on sperm parameters of males suffering from sub fertility related to low sperm quality.* **Siterman, S, et al.,** 1997, Arch Androl, pp. 155-61.

293. *Does acupuncture treatment affect sperm density in males with very low sperm count? A pilot study.* **Siterman, S, et al.,** s.l. : Andrologia, 2000, Vol. 32.

294. *Effects of acupuncture and moxa treatment in patients with semen abnormalities.* **Gurfinkel, Edson , et al.,** s.l. : Asian J Androl, 2003, Vol. 5.

295. *Point- and frequency-specific response of the testicular artery to abdominal electroacupuncture in humans.* **Cakmak, Y, et al.,** 5, s.l. : Fertility and Sterility, 2008, Vol. 90.

296. *Quantitative evaluation of spermatozoa ultrastructure after acupuncture treatment for idiopathic male infertility.* **Pei, J, et al.,** 1, s.l. : Fertility and Sterility, 2005, Vol. 84.

297. *Success of acupuncture treatment in patients with initially low sperm output is associated with a decrease in scrotal skin temperature.* **Siterman, Shimon , et al.,** s.l. : Asian Journal of Andrology, 2009.

298. *Effect of electro-acupuncture stimulation of different frequencies and intensities on ovarian blood flow in anaesthetized rats with steroid-induced polycystic ovaries.* **Stener-Victorin, Elisabet , et al.,** 16, s.l. : Reproductive Biology and Endocrinology, 2004, Vol. 2.

299. *Electroacupuncture reduces uterine artery blood flow impedance in infertile women.* **Ming, Ho, et al.,** 2, s.l. : Taiwan J Obstet Gynecol, 2009, Vol. 48.

300. *Ovarian blood flow responses to electroacupuncture stimulation depend on estrous cycle and on site and frequency of stimulation in anesthetized rats.* **Stener-Victorin, Elisabet , Fujisawa, Shigeko and Kurosawa, Mieko .** s.l. : J Appl Physiol, 2006, Vol. 101.

301. *Effects of Acupuncture on Anxiety Levels and Prefrontal Cortex Activity Measured by Near-Infrared Spectroscopy: A Pilot Study.* **Sakatani, K, et al.,** s.l. : Adv Exp Med Biol, 2016.

302. *The relationship between perceived stress, acupuncture, and pregnancy rates among IVF patients: a pilot study.* **Balk, J, et al.,** s.l. : Complementary Therapies in Clinical Practice, 2010.

303. *The effect of acupuncture on uterine contraction induced by oxytocin.* **Pak, S, et al.,** 1, s.l. : Am J Chin Med, 2000, Vol. 28.

304. *Effect of acupuncture treatment on uterine motility and cyclooxygenase-2 expression in pregnant rats.* **Kim, J, Shin, K and Na, C.** 4, s.l. : Gynecol Obstet Invest, 2000, Vol. 50.

305. *Enhancement of splenic interferon-gamma, interleukin-2, and NK cytotoxicity by S36 acupoint acupuncture in F344 rats.* **Yu, Y, et al.,** s.l. : Japanese Journal of Physiology, 1997, Vol. 47.

306. *Acupuncture Regulates Leukocyte Subpopulations in Human Peripheral Blood.* **Yamaguchi, Nobuo , et al.,** 4, s.l. : Evidence Based Complementary Alternative Medicine, 2007, Vol. 4.

307. *Anti-inflammatory actions of acupuncture.* **Zijlstra, Freek, et al.,** 2, s.l. : Mediators of Inflammation, 2003, Vol. 12.

308. *Antipyretic effects of acupuncture on the lipopolysaccharideinduced fever and expression of interleukin-6 and interleukin-1b mRNAs in the hypothalamus of rats.* **Son, Yang-Sun, et al.,** s.l. : Neuroscience Letters, 2002, Vol. 319.

309. *Electro-acupuncture at Acupoint ST36 Ameliorates Inflammation and Regulates Th1/Th2 Balance in Delayed-Type Hypersensitivity.* **Wang, Zhigang , et al.,** s.l. : Inflammation, 2016.

310. *Effect of Acupuncture on Infertility Due to Luteal Phase Defect.* **Yang , Hong-wei and Huang , Xue-yan .** 2, s.l. : J. Acupunct. Tuina. Sci, 2012, Vol. 10.

311. *Compounds of Natural Origin and Acupuncture for the Treatment of Diseases Caused by Estrogen Deficiency.* **Thakur, A, Mandal, S and Banerjee, S.** 3, s.l. : Journal of Acupuncture and Meridian Studies, 2016, Vol. 9.

312. *Clinical studies on the mechanism for acupuncture stimulation of ovulation.* **Mo, X, et al.,** 2, s.l. : J Tradit Chin Med, 1993, J Tradit Chin Med, Vol. 13, pp. 115-9.

313. *One hundred years of aspirin.* **Jack, David.** s.l. : The Lancet, 1997, Vol. 350.

314. **Wilson, Edward.** *The Diversity Of Life.* s.l. : The Belknap Press Of Harvard University Press, 1993.

315. *Effects of Bushen Tiaochong Recipe (补肾调冲方) Containing Serum on Ovarian Granulosa Cell Proliferation, Steroidogenesis and Associated Gene Expression in Rats.* **Xia, T, et al.,** s.l. : Chin J Integr Med, 2007, Vol. 3.

316. *Eighty-seven cases of male infertility treated by bushen shengjing pill in clinical observation and evaluation on its curative effect.* **Yue, G P, Chen, Q and Dai, N.** 8, s.l. : Chung Kuo Chung Hsi I Chieh Ho Tsa Chih, 1996, Vol. 16.

317. *Direct effects of Chinese herbal medicine "hachuekkito" on sperm movement.* **Yamanaka, M, et al.,** 1998, Nippon Hinyokika Gakkai Zasshi, pp. 641-6.

318. *Effects of guizhi-fuling-wan on male infertility with varicocele.* **Ishikawa, H, et al.,** s.l. : Am J Chin Med, 1996, Am J Chin Med, Vol. 24, pp. 327-31.

319. *Improvements in Scrotal Thermoregulation in Patients with Varicoceles Treated by Using Traditional Korean Medicine: Two Case Reports.* **Jo, J, Kim, H and Jerng, U.** s.l. : J Acupunct Meridian Stud, 2016.

320. *Wen-Jing-Tang, a Traditional Chinese Herbal Medicine Increases Luteinizing Hormone Release In Vitro.* **Miyake, Akira , et al.,** s.l. : The American Journal of Chinese Medicine, 1986, Vol. 14.

321. *Effect of soothing liver therapy on oocyte quality and growth differentiation factor-9 in patients undergoing in vitro fertilization and embry ot ransfer.* **Gao, Xing, et al.,** 5, s.l. : J Tradit Chin Med, 2013, Vol. 33.

322. *A substance isolated from Cornus officinalis enhances the motility of human sperm.* **Jeng, H, et al.,** 1997, Am J Chin Med, pp. 3-4.

323. *The Relationship between Traditional Chinese Medicine and Modern Medicine.* **Dong, Jingcheng .** s.l. : Evidence-Based Complementary and Alternative Medicine, 2013.

324. *Prevalance And Economic Burden Of Medication Errors In The NHS In England.* **Elliot, Rachel, et al.,** s.l. : Policy Research Unit in Economic Evaluation of Health & Care Interventions (EEPRU), 2018.

325. **Williams, Steven .** *Health and social care directorate.* s.l. : National Institute of

Health and Care Excellence, 2015.

326. *Medical error—the third leading cause of death in the US.* **Makary, Martin and Daniel, Michael** . s.l. : BMJ, 2016.

327. *Uterine glandular area during the menstrual cycle and the effects of different in-vitro fertilization related hormonal treatments.* **Rogers, P, et al.**, 2, s.l. : Human Reproduction, 1996, Vol. 11.

328. *Polycystic Ovary Syndrome: Effect and Mechanisms of Acupuncture for Ovulation Induction.* **Johansson, Julia and Stener-Victorin, Elisabet.** s.l. : Evidence-Based Complementary and Alternative Medicine, 2013.

329. *Use of clomiphene citrate and birth defects, National Birth Defects Prevention Study, 1997–2005.* **Reefhuis, J, et al.**, 2, Atlanta : Human Reproduction, 2011, Vol. 26.

330. *Acupuncture and Chinese herbal treatment for women undergoing intrauterine insemination.* **Sela, Keren, et al.**, s.l. : European Journal of Integrative Medicine, 2011.

331. *Risk Assessment of Using Aluminum Foil in Food Preparation.* **Bassioni, Ghada. et al.** Int. J. Electrochem. Sci., 7 (2012) 4498 - 4509.

332. *Coenzyme Q10 and Statin-Induced Mitochondrial Dysfunction.* **Deichmann, Richard, et al.** The Ochsner Journal 10:16–21, 2010.

333. *Treatment of statin adverse effects with supplemental Coenzyme Q10 and statin drug discontinuation.* **Langsjoen, Peter, et al.** BioFactors 25 (2005) 147–152.

334. *Muscle Coenzyme Q10 Level in Statin-Related Myopathy.* **Lamperti, Costanza, et al.** Arch Neurol. 2005; 62: 1709-1712.

335. *Ginseng, the 'Immunity Boost': The Effects of Panax ginseng on Immune System.* **Kang, Soowon, et al.** J Ginseng Res Vol. 2012; 36, No. 4, 354-368.

336. *Ginsenoside Rg1 enhances CD4(+) T-cell activities and modulates Th1/Th2 differentiation.* **Lee, E, et al.** Int Immunopharmacol 2004; 4: 235-244.

337. *Acupuncture Increases Nocturnal Melatonin Secretion and Reduces Insomnia and Anxiety: A Preliminary Report.* **D, Warren Spence, et al.** J Neuropsychiatry Clin Neurosci 2004; 16, 1.

338. *Hormones in international meat production: biological,sociological and consumer issues.* **Galbraith, H.** Nutrition Research Reviews 2002, 15: 293–314.

339. *Phthalates: European regulation, chemistry, pharmacokinetic and related toxicity.* **Ventrice, P, et al.** Environmental toxicology and pharmacology 2013: 3, 6: 88–96.

340. *Autism genes are selectively targeted by environmental pollutants including pesticides, heavy metals, bisphenol A, phthalates and many others in food, cosmetics or household products.* **Carter, C, et al.** Neurochemistry International 2016; 101: 83-109.

341. *Increased Serum Phthalates (MEHP, DEHP) and Bisphenol A Concentrations in Children With Autism Spectrum Disorder: The Role of Endocrine Disruptors in Autism Etiopathogenesis.* **Kardas, F, et al.** Journal of Child Neurology 2015.

342. **Wiseman, Nigel.** *A Practical Dictionary of Chinese Medicine.* Brookline: Paradigm Publications, 1998.

343. *Effect of a vegetarian diet and dexamethasone on plasma prolactin, testosterone and dehydroepiandrosterone in men and women.* **Hill, P, et al.** Cancer Letters 1979; 7, No. 5, 273-282.

344. *Diet and Reproductive Hormones: A Study of Vegetarian and Nonvegetarian Postmenopausal Women.* **Armstrong, B, et al.** Journal of the National Cancer Institute 1981; 67; No. 4. 761–767.

345. *Effect of dietary components, including lignans and phytoestrogens, on enterohepatic circulation and liver metabolism of estrogens and on sex hormone binding globulin (SHBG).* **Adlercreutz, H, et al.** Journal of Steroid Biochemistry 1987; 27, No. 4–6, 1135-1144.

346. *Association of coffee, green tea, and caffeine intakes with serum concentrations of estradiol and sex hormone-binding globulin in premenopausal Japanese women.* **Nagata, C, et al.** Nutrition and Cancer 1998; 30, No. 1, 21-24.

347. *Glyphosate Use Predicts Healthcare Utilization for ADHD in the Healthcare Cost and Utilization Project net (HCUPnet): A Two-Way Fixed-Effects Analysis.* **Fluegge, K, et al.** 2016: Pol. J. Environ. Stud. Vol. 25; No. 4, 1489-1503.

348. *Allergies, asthma, ADHD: Is it the food we eat?* **Peper, E.** 2015. Research Gate:

https://www.researchgate.net/publication/277019795.

349. *Glyphosate's Suppression of Cytochrome P450 Enzymes and Amino Acid Biosynthesis by the Gut Microbiome: Pathways to Modern Diseases.* **Samsel A, et al.** 2013: Entropy 15: 1417-1463.

350. *The Possible Link between Autism and Glyphosate Acting as Glycine Mimetic - A Review of Evidence from the Literature with Analysis.* **Beecham, J, et al.** J Mol Genet Med 2015; 9; No. 4.

351. *Environmental factors in the development of autism spectrum disorders.* **Sealey, L, et al.** Environment International 2016; 88, 288–298.

352. *Aluminum and Glyphosate Can Synergistically Induce Pineal Gland Pathology: Connection to Gut Dysbiosis and Neurological Disease.* **Seneff, S, et al.** Agricultural Sciences 2015; 6, 42-70.

353. *A comparison of temporal trends in United States autism prevalence to trends in suspected environmental factors.* **Nevison, C.** Nevison Environmental Health 2014; 13, 73.

354. *Activation of the epithelial Na+ channel triggers prostaglandin E2 release and production required for embryo implantation.* **Ruan, Y, et al.** Nature Medicine 2012; 18, 1112–1117.

355. *Human cumulus granulosa cell gene expression: a predictor of fertilization and embryo selection in women undergoing IVF.* **McKenzie, L, et al.** Human Reproduction 2004; 19; No.12, 2869–2874.

356. *Characterization of the Sperm Proteome and Reproductive Outcomes with in Vitro Fertilization after a Reduction in Male Ejaculatory Abstinence Period.* **Shen Z, et al.** Molecular & Cellular Proteomics March 15, 2019.

357. *Electroacupuncture Facilitates Implantation by Enhancing Endometrial Angiogenesis in a Rat Model of Ovarian Hyperstimulation.* **Chen, W, et al.** Biology of Reproduction, Volume 100, Issue 1, January 2019, Pages 268–280.

358. *NAD+ Repletion Rescues Female Fertility during Reproductive Aging.* **Bertoldo, M, et al.** 2020, Cell Reports 30, 1670–1681.

Index

antioxidants **72-4**, 131, 160, 163, 180, 186, 190, 192, 193, 195, 196, 197

antral follicle count (AFC) 35, **50-1**, 146, 188, 206;
testing 50

anxiety 21, 28, 55, 57, **74-5**, 88, 90, 92, 96, 97, 100, 110, 112, 120, 134, 135, 136, 138, 151, 157, 162, 206;
see also stress response

apigenin **172**, 173, 175, 193

attention deficit hyperactivity disorder (ADHD) 62

autism 21, 62, 63, 64, 68, 71, 144, 151, 189, 190

B

baths versus showers 121-2

B cells 52, **53**

bee pollen 175, **186**

beta-carotene 73, 173, **186**, 188, 192, 195

biotin 186

birth defects 47, 51, 73, 105, 146, 147, 148, 151, 188, 189, 195, 196, 215-6;
see also chromosome abnormalities

bisphenol A (BPA) **64**, 144-5

bisphenol S (BPS) 64

blood 84-6; donating 126

blood clot *see* thrombophilia test

blood deficiency 90-3;

causes 92
risks 92-3
symptoms 90-1
testing 91
treatment 93

blood stasis 98-100;
causes 98-9
risks 99
symptoms 98
testing 98
treatment 99-100

body temperature **40-1**, 85, 100, 103, 111, 113, 114, 122, 124, 125, 146;
see also charting

bromelain **186-7**, 195

C

cadmium (Cd) 130, 131, **147-8**

caffeine 88, 89, 90, 93, 111, 130, 159, **167**, 187, 190, 191, 195

calcium 23, 131, 148, 167, **187**, 190, 194, 197

carbohydrates 20, 33, 130, 131, 159, 160, **165**, 175

cervical mucus **39**, 42 (figure), 43, 58, 78, 80, 81, 169

charting 40-1

chemicals 34, 56, **59-69**, 141-2, 143, 168, 170, 174
reducing exposure to 141-2

Chinese herbs Ch 14;

Printed in Great Britain
by Amazon

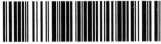